Cheers for Brave Like Me!

"The whole book is good! And it helps you be safe and healthy."

Makenzie S., Age 7

"I am so in love with this story! This book safely explains coronavirus to children and gives them preventative measures they can easily follow. It also gives our children coping skills to manage their anxieties during the pandemic! I highly recommend this book to all parents and educators of young children!"

Maia Bean
Professional School Counselor

"This book is such a family friendly reading essential. And the content is helpful for families beyond the coronavirus because it can be used as an informational resource. Having the correct information also helps to minimize fear, especially in children, and provides the opportunity for questions. This type of content can also help encourage a new generation of public health leaders."

Leola Griffin
Mom and Clinical Research Professional

"The year 2020 has been a remarkable year in many ways. New words, or rarely used words and phrases like pandemic, contact tracing, and social distancing are now common vernacular. New habits and changes in behavior...all of which stresses the human form and community. Children sense these changes and pick up that tension. Tickles and Rona are lovely characters who work through these troubled times in a collaborative way which a child can understand. Resisting fear and anxiety with facts is good therapy, and Ms. Beckett has done just that with this children's story. I highly recommend it"

Charlie Howsare, MD, MPH
Physician and Public Health Consultant

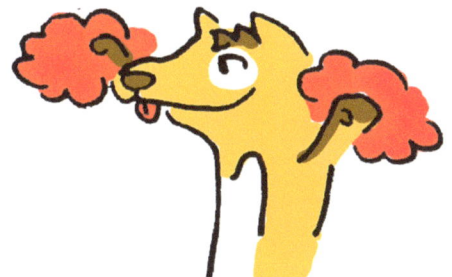

Brave Like Me!

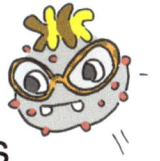

Courageous Lessons About the COVID-19 Coronavirus and Healthy Coping for Children and Families Anytime

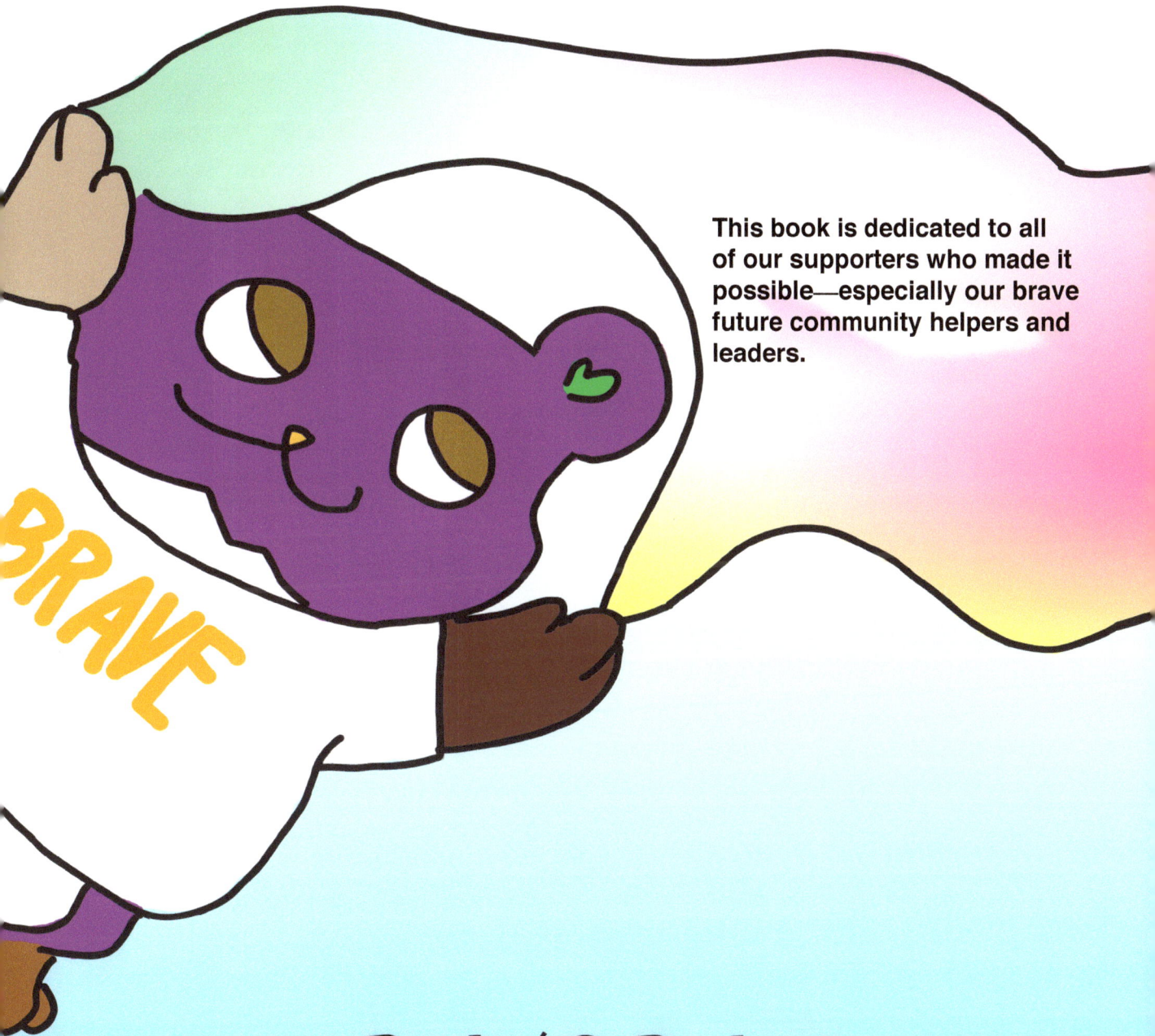

This book is dedicated to all of our supporters who made it possible—especially our brave future community helpers and leaders.

BRAVE

Donica G. Beckett

Brave Like Me!

Courageous Lessons About the COVID-19 Coronavirus
and Healthy Coping for Children and Families Anytime

Author:

Donica' G. Beckett

https://completepackagepub.com

Illustrator & Cover Designer:

Jean Marie Munson

https://plottwistpublishing.com

Editor:

Connie B. Dowell

https://bookechoes.com

Spanish Translator:

Elizabeth Bobo

https://linkedin.com/in/elizabethgbobo

Paperback ISBN: 978-1-7367107-0-8   Hardback ISBN: 978-1-7367107-1-5

Library of Congress Control Number: 2021903632

COMPLETE PACKAGE
— P U B L I S H I N G —
& C O M M U N I C A T I O N S

Complete Package Publishing and Communications, LLC ♥ Houston, Texas, USA

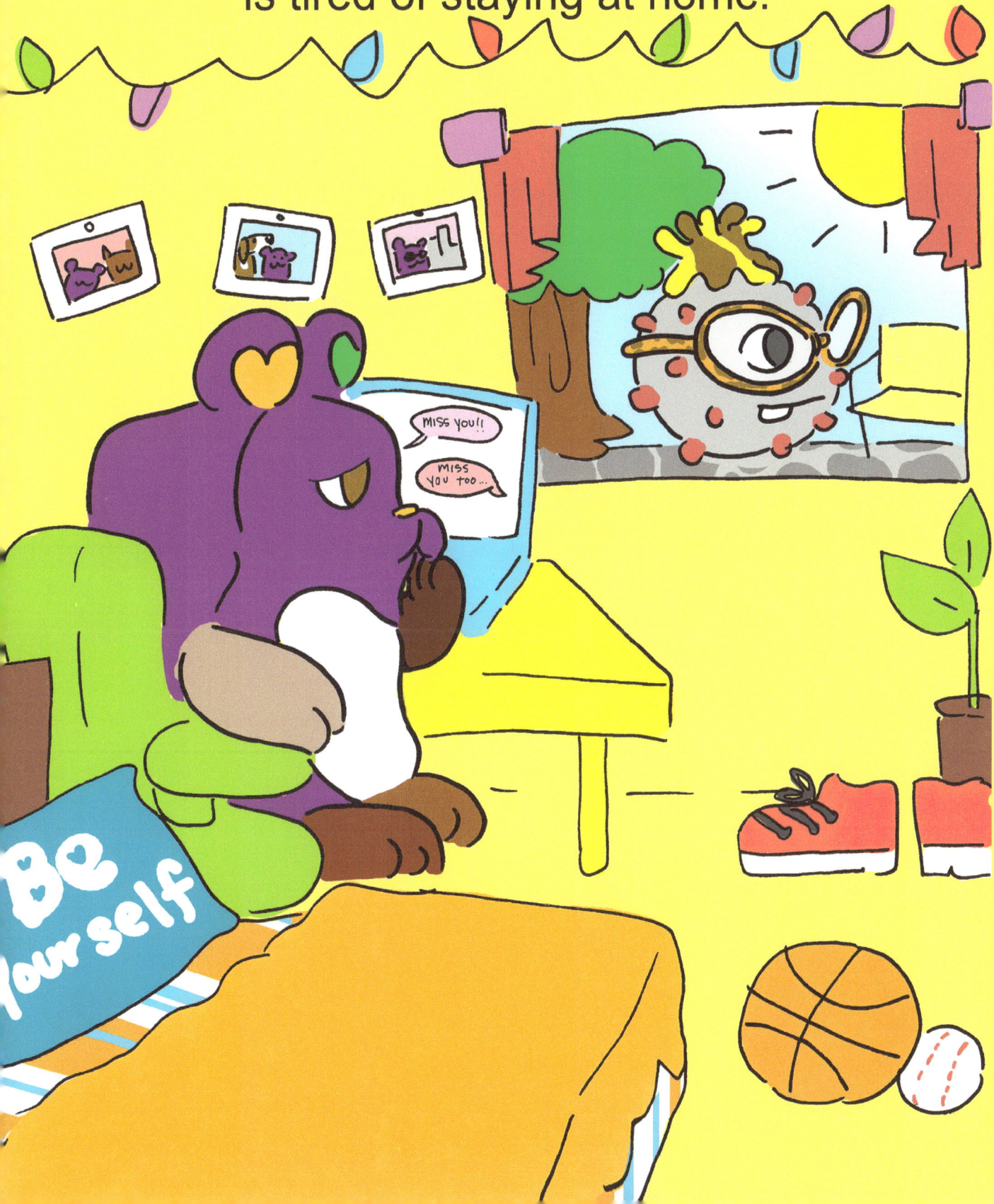

Tickles the Brave Teddy™
is tired of staying at home.

Tickles misses friends at school, wants to play, and find out what's going on.

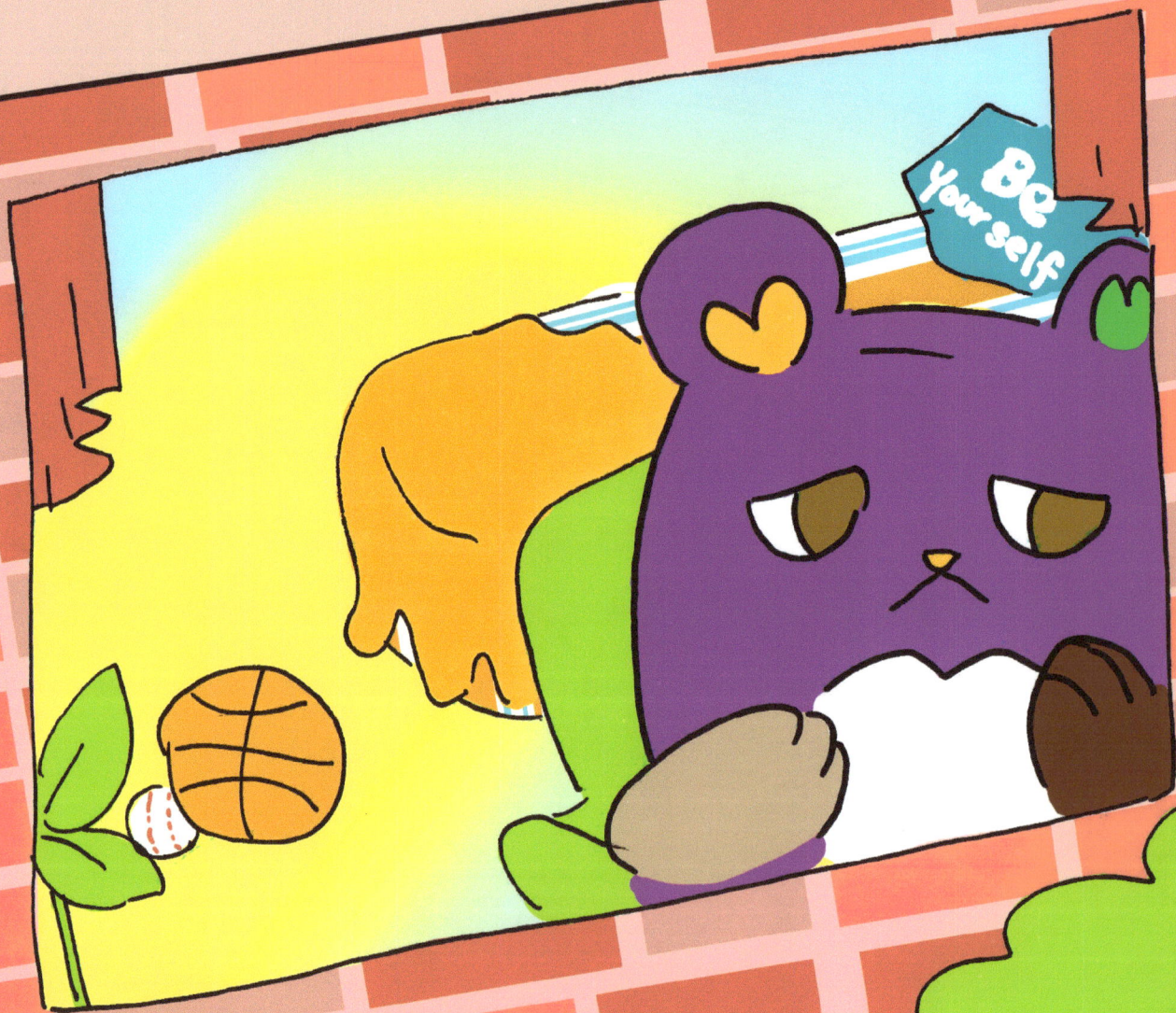

"Hi, my name is Tickles.
What's your name? Do you want to play?"

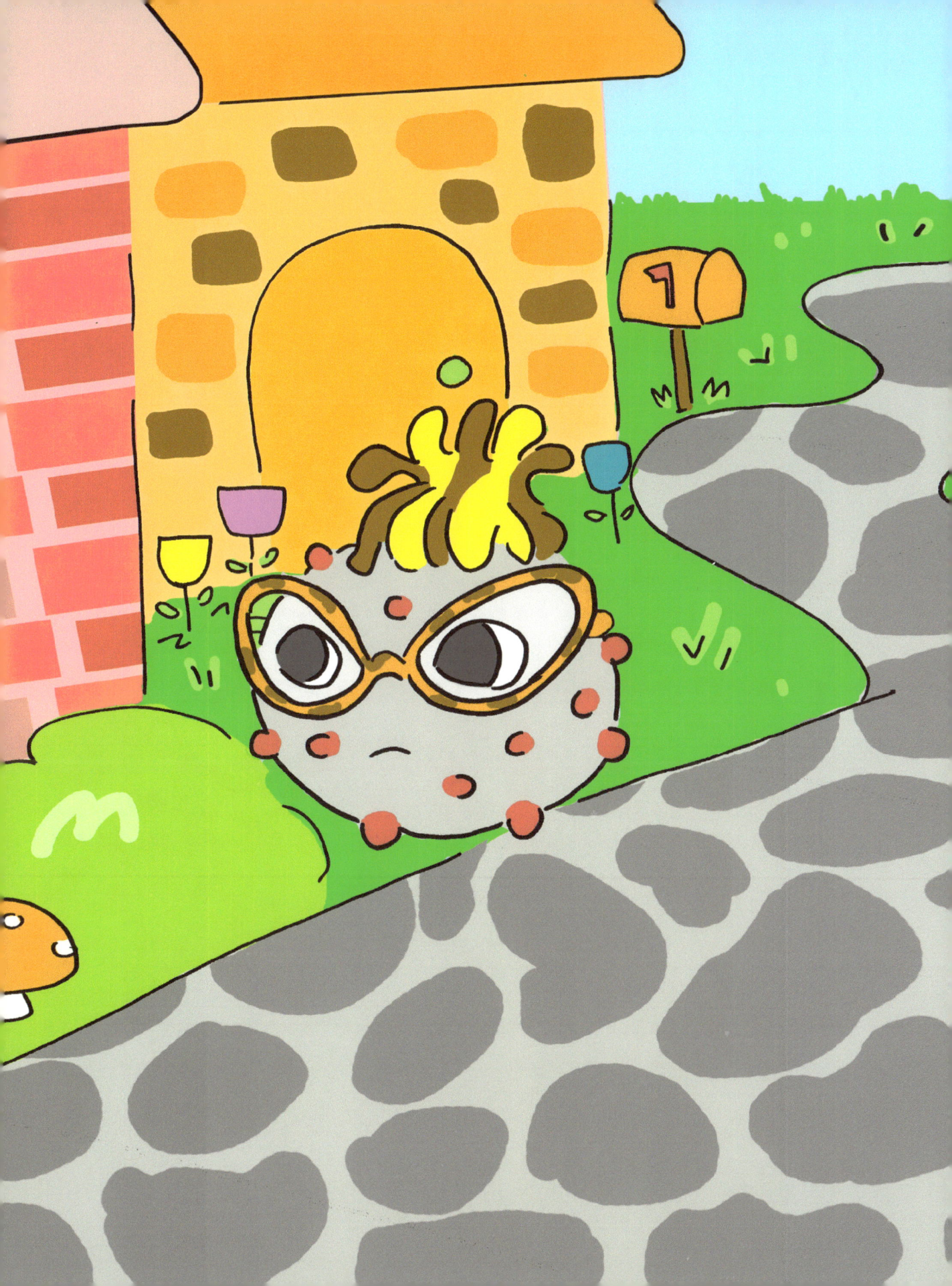

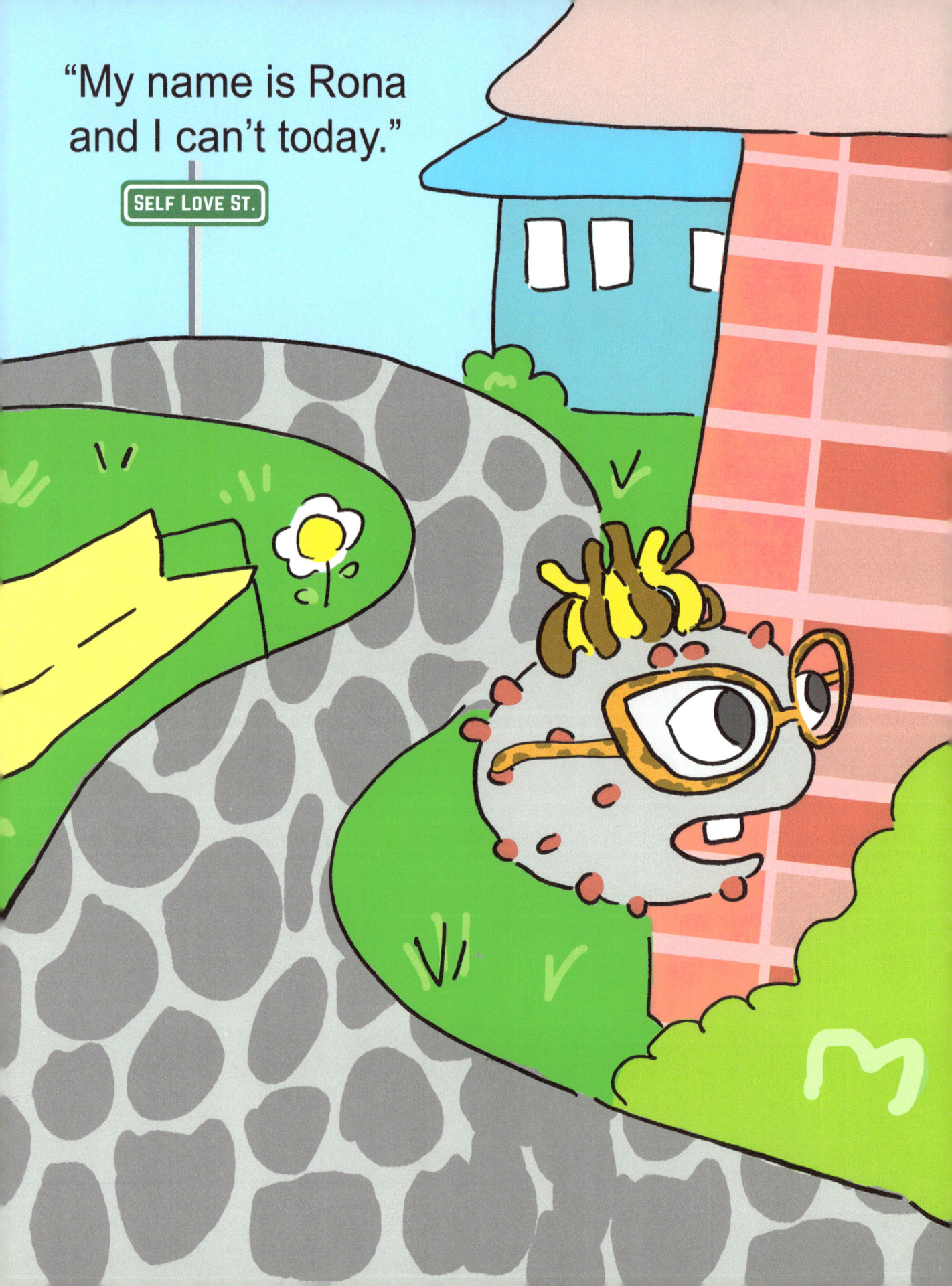

"Why, Rona? Look at the sky. It's not gray."

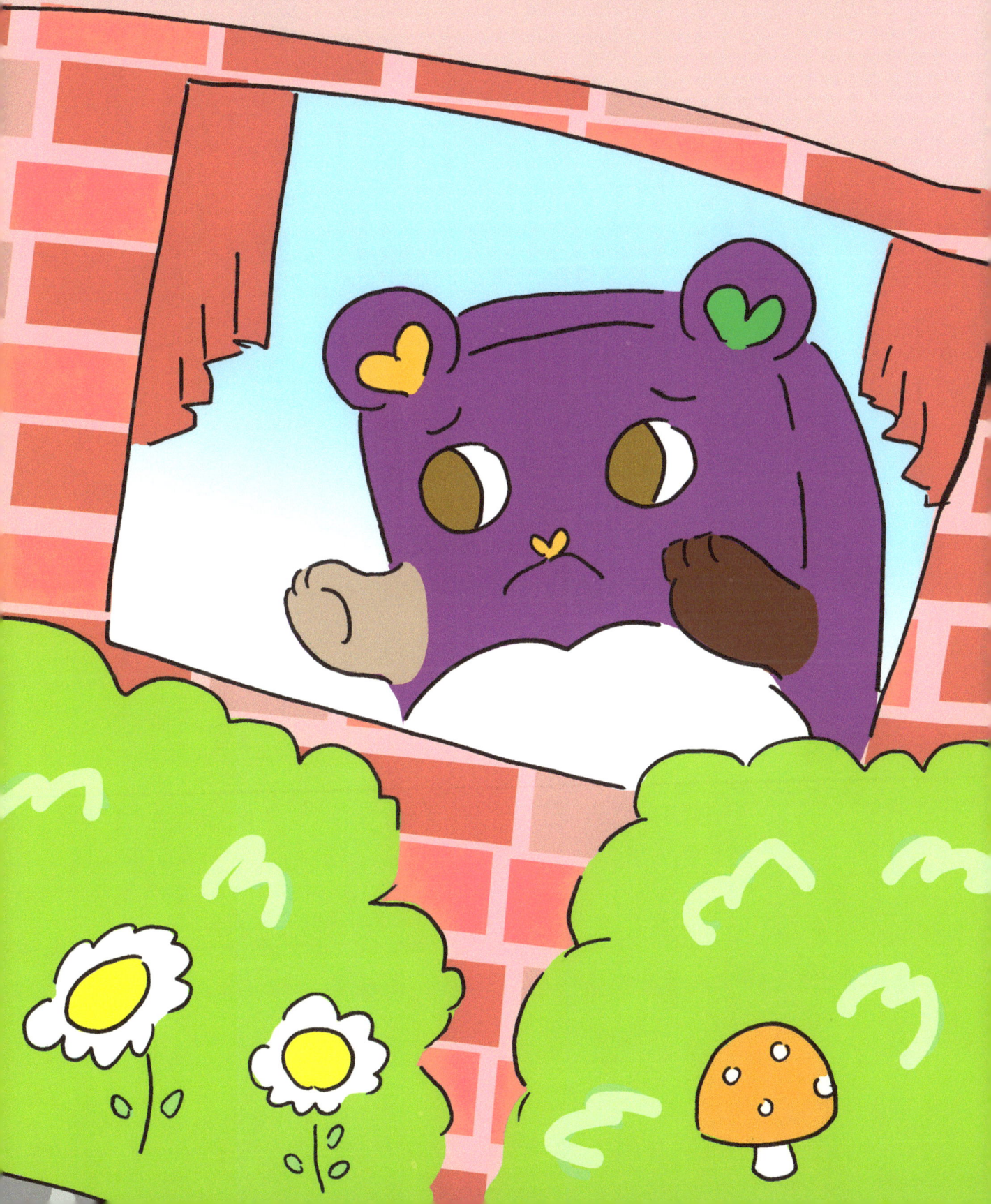

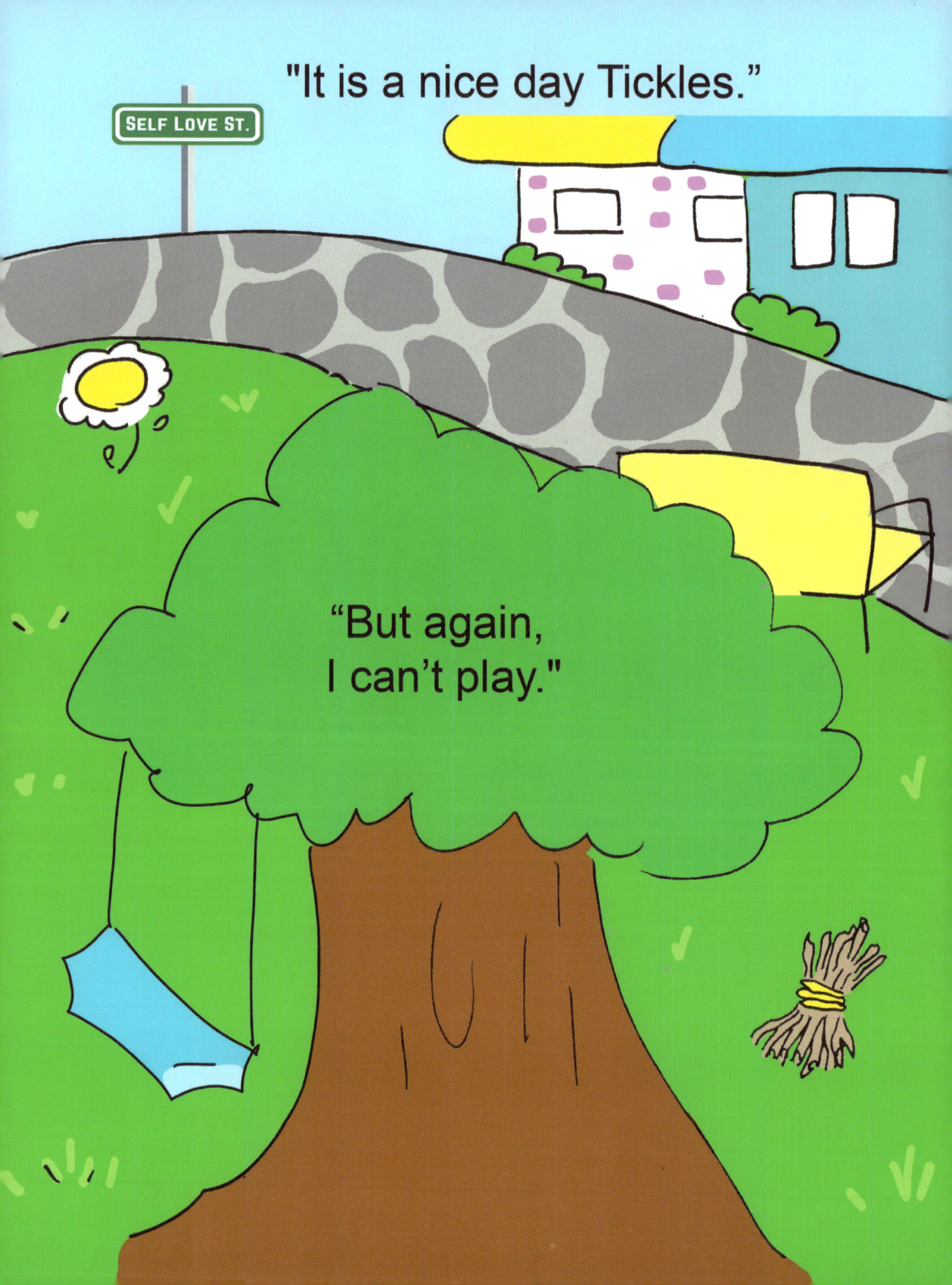

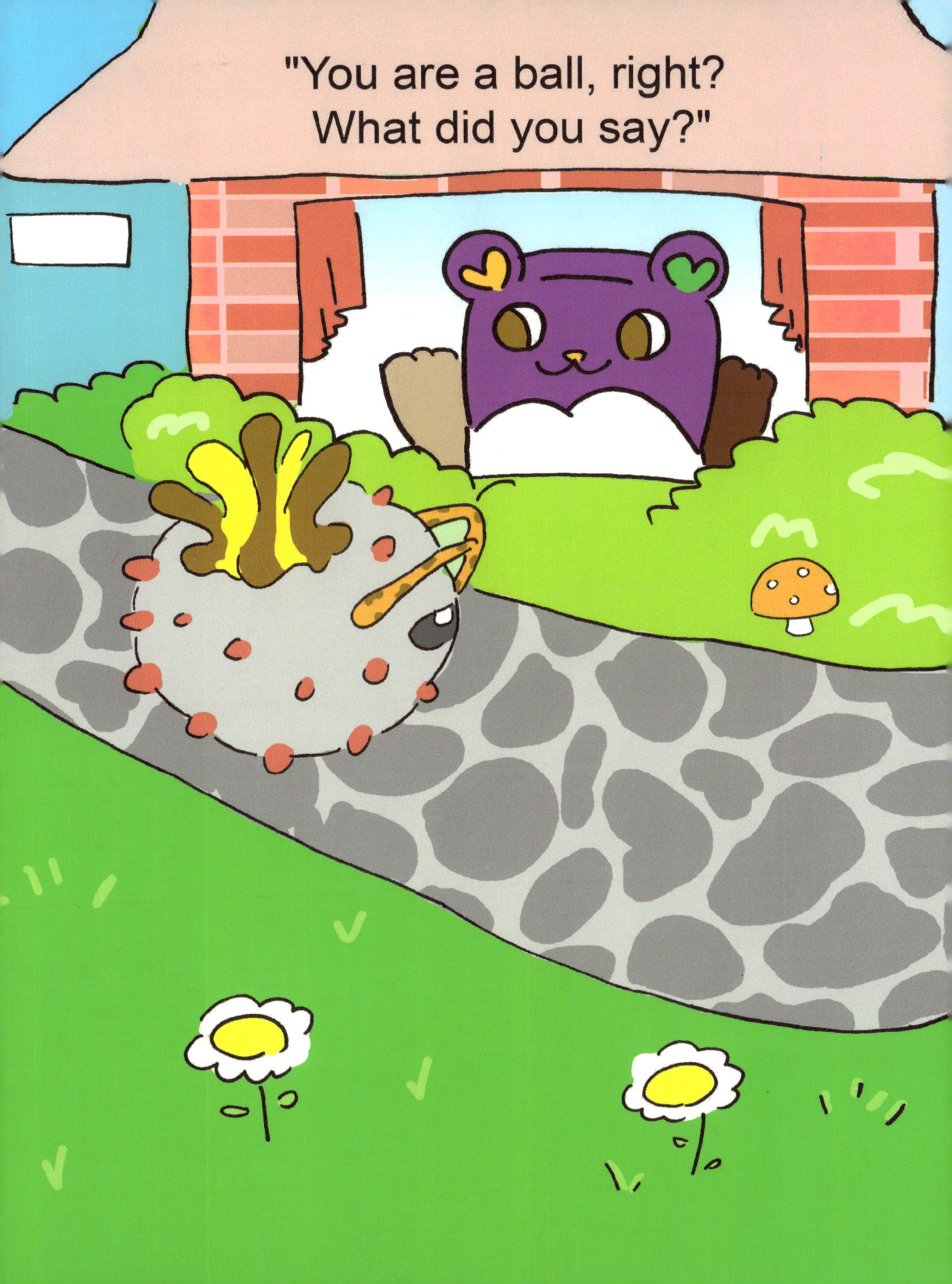

"You are a ball, right?
What did you say?"

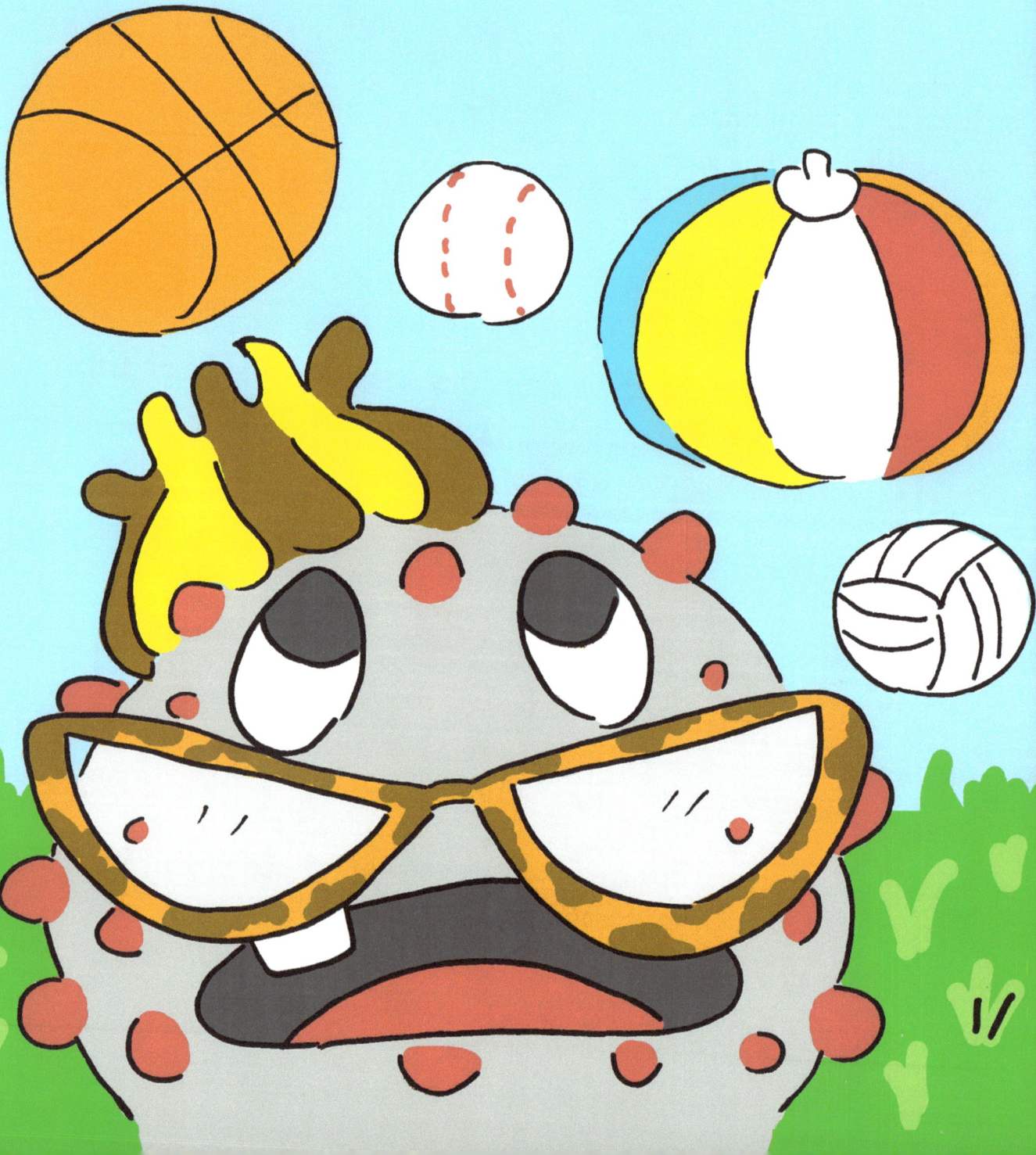

"I'm not like any ball you have ever seen.
I could make you sick if you play with me."

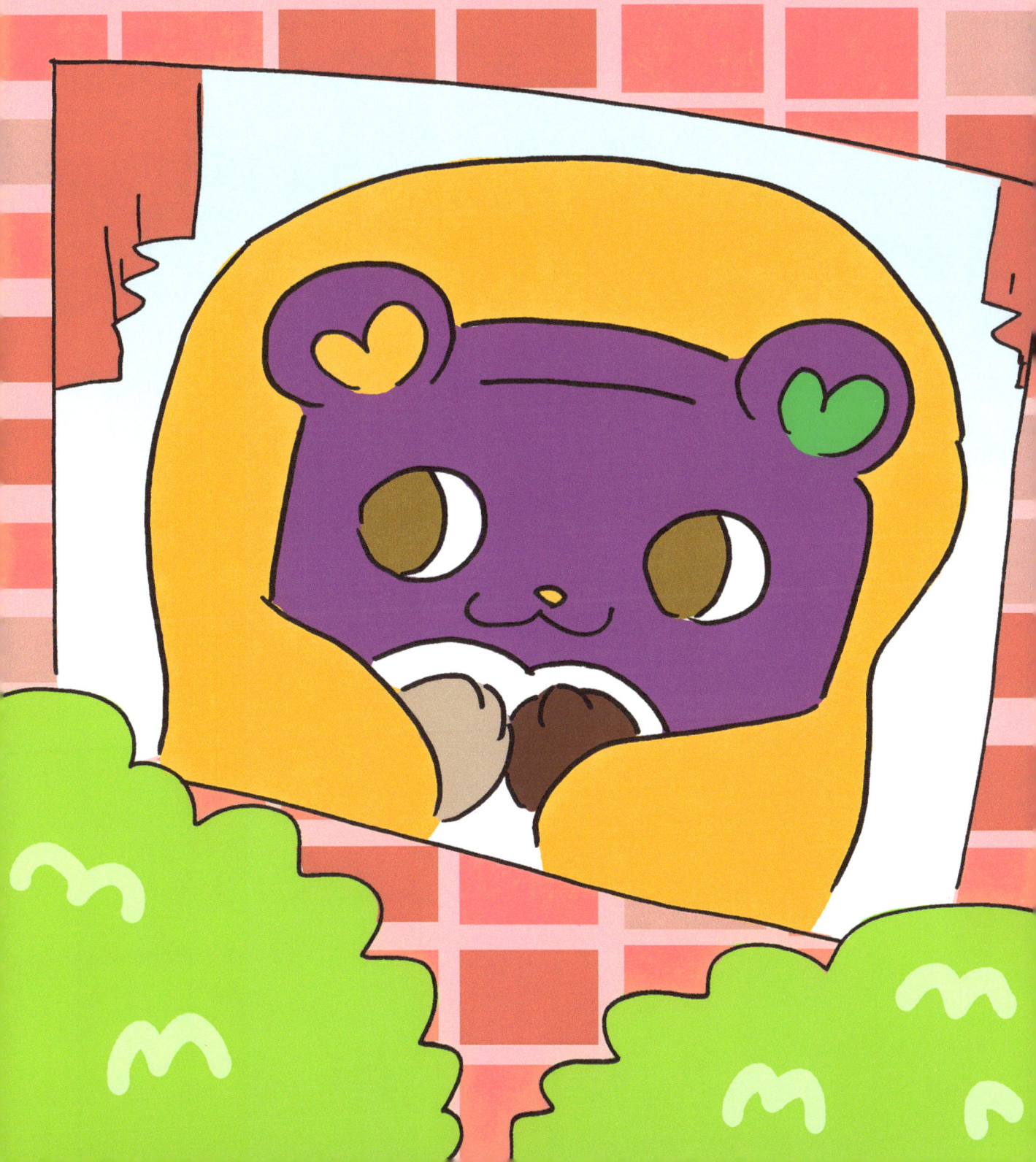

"How could that be? I do not want to get sick."

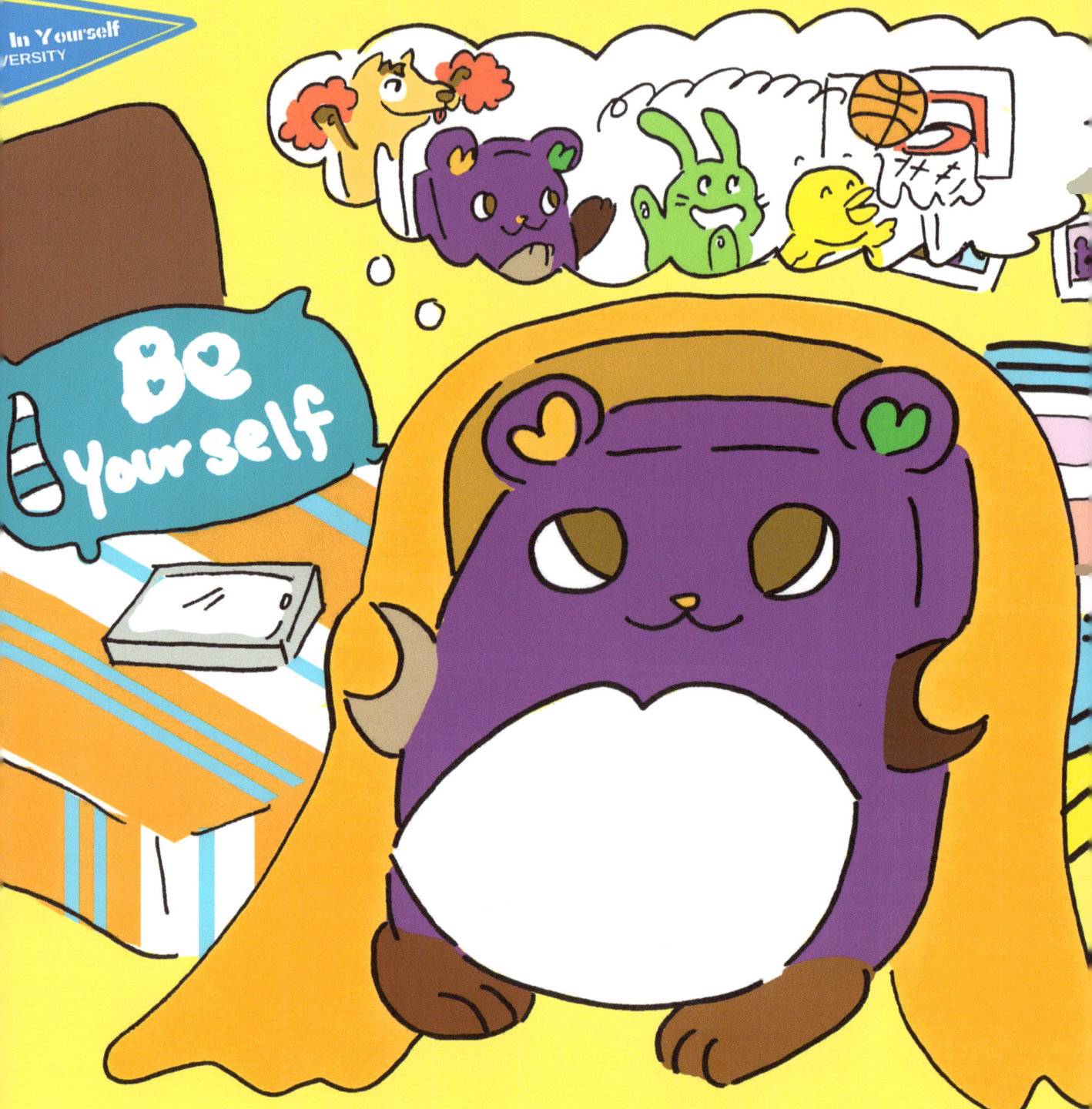

"I know you miss your friends and want to play, but let me teach you why this is not a trick."

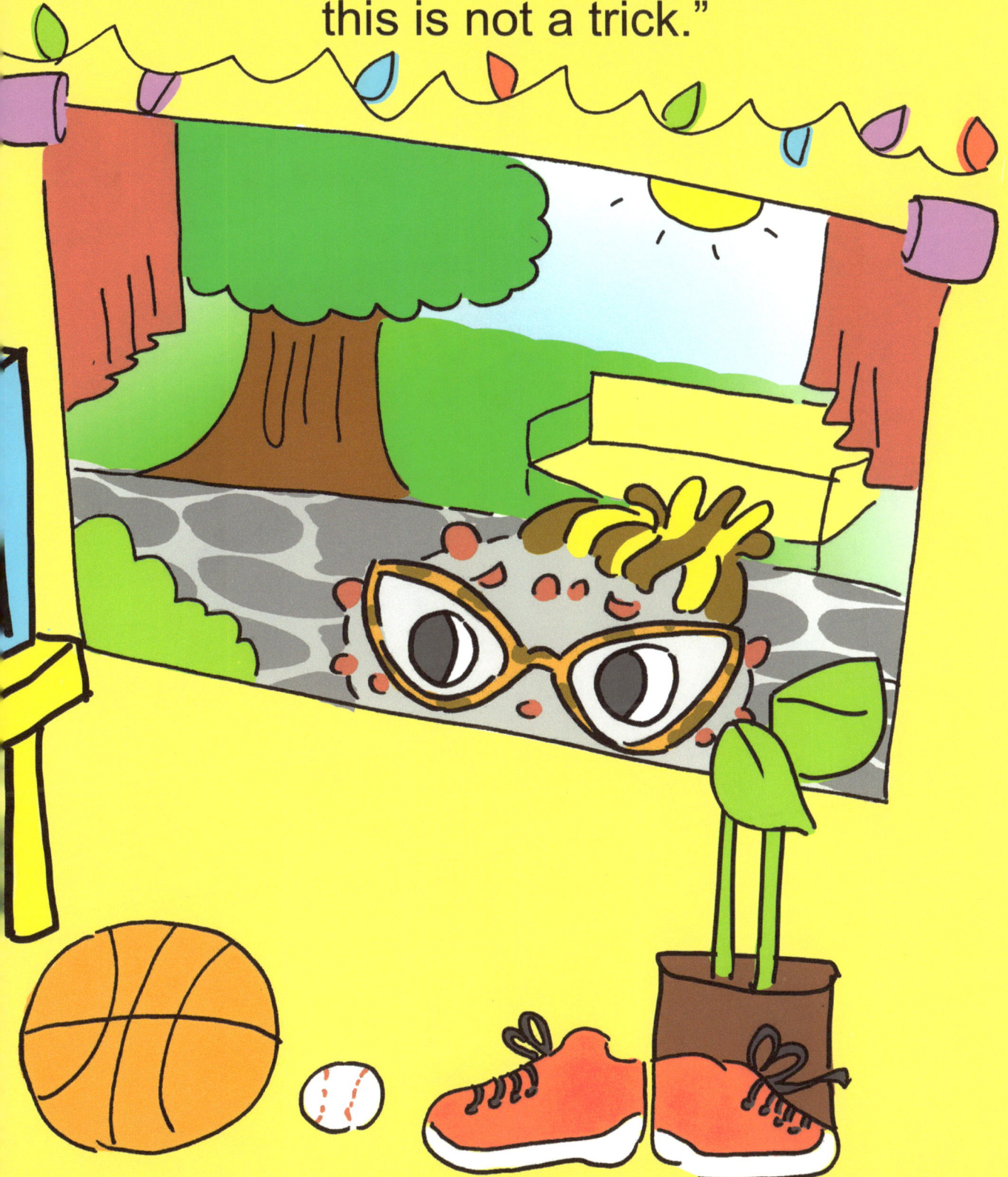

"Listen up really quick.
My real name is COVID-19, and I come from
a large family called coronavirus.
Some people call me Rona for short."

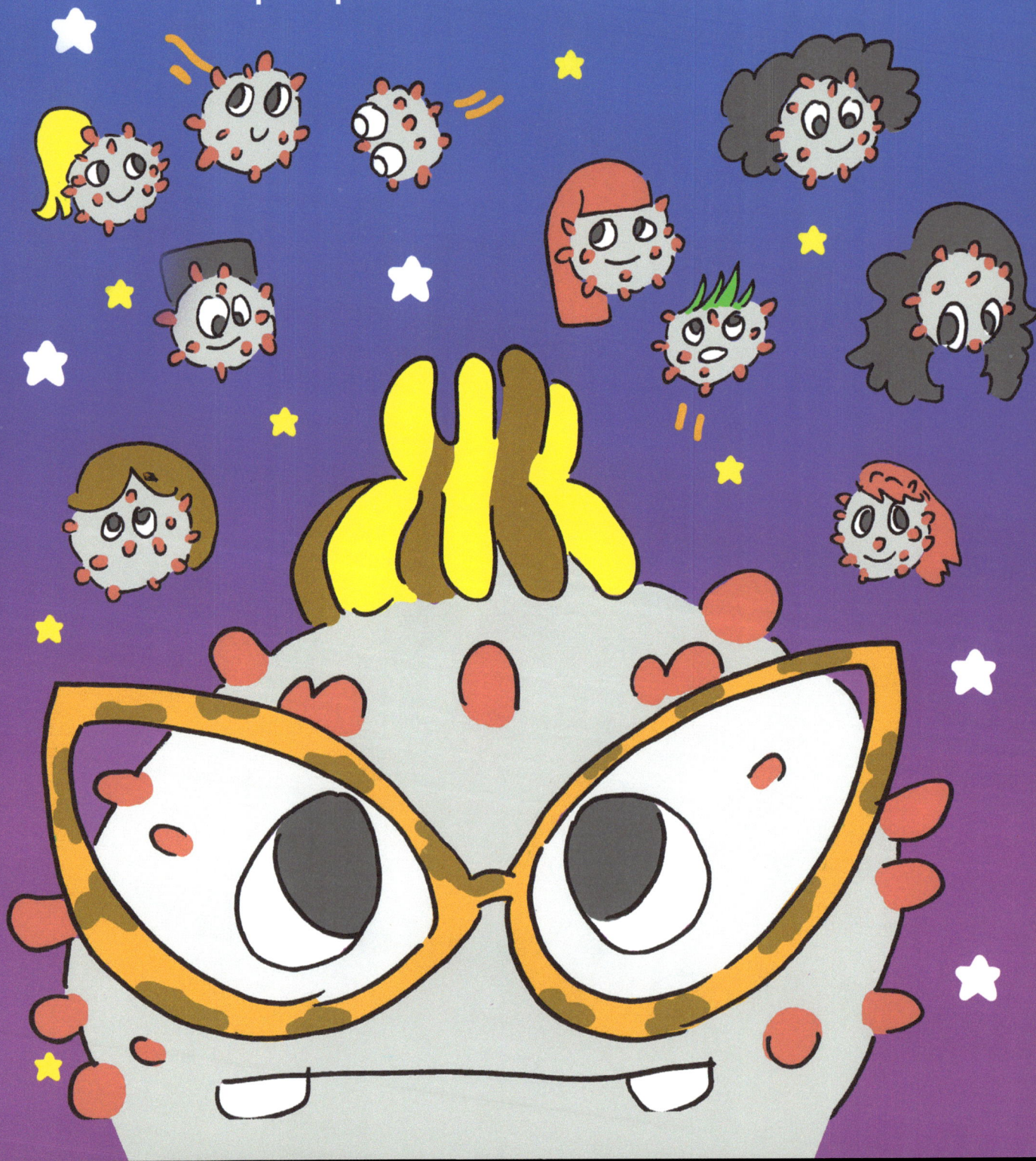

"Like in sports, tons of 'balls' that look just like me bounce all around the world."

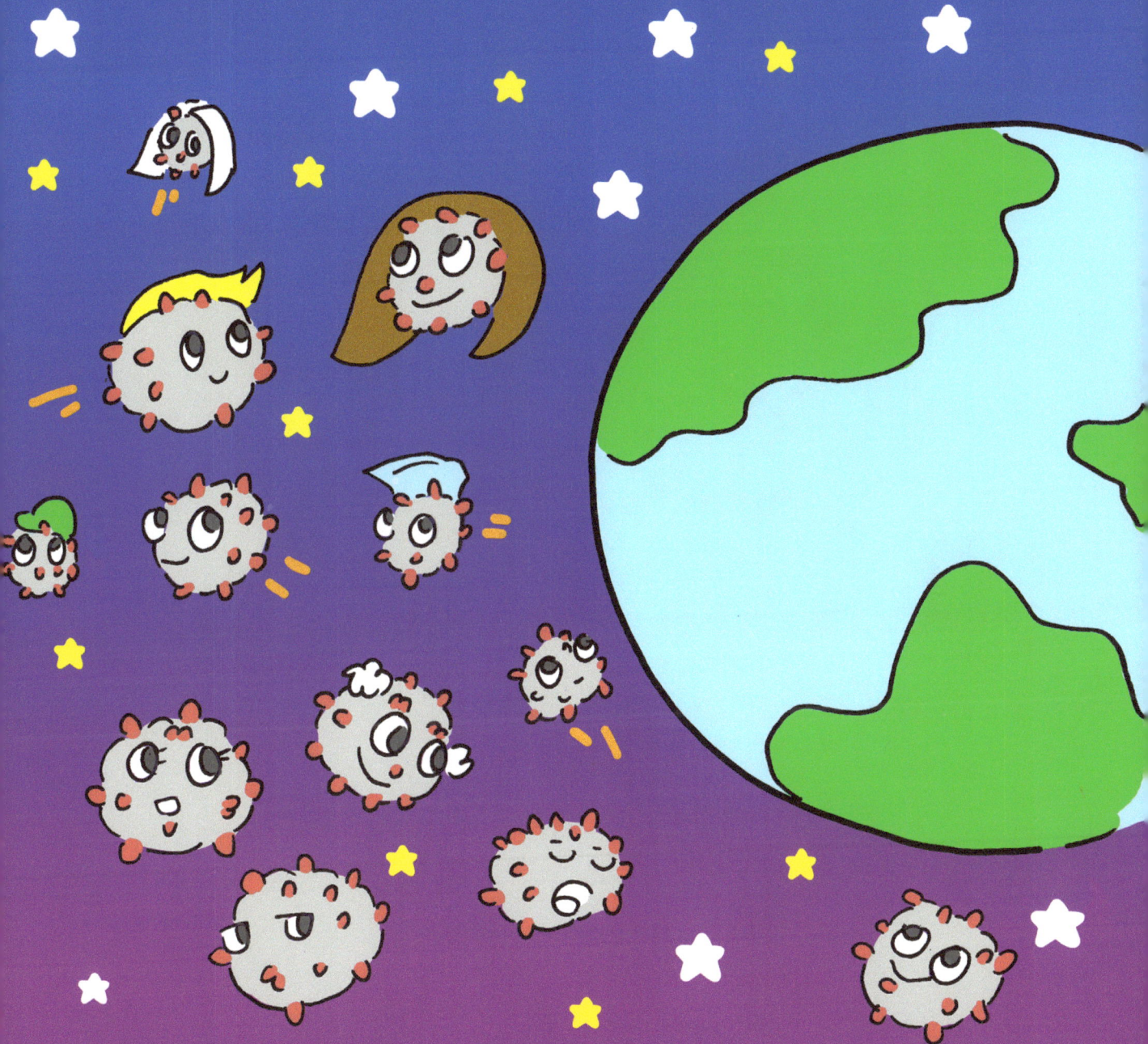

"I can be found in over 200 places:
The United States, Spain,
Italy, and many more."

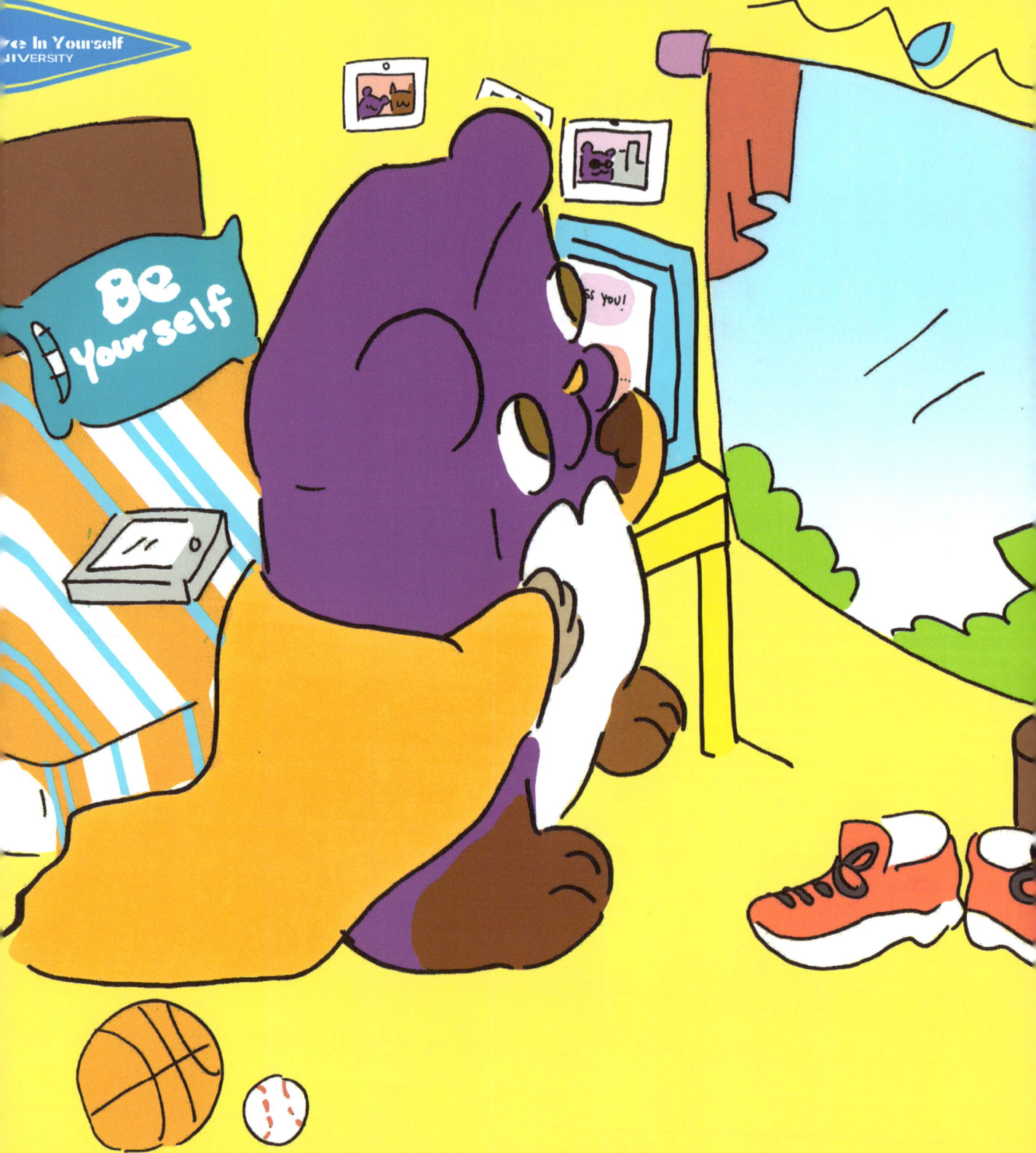

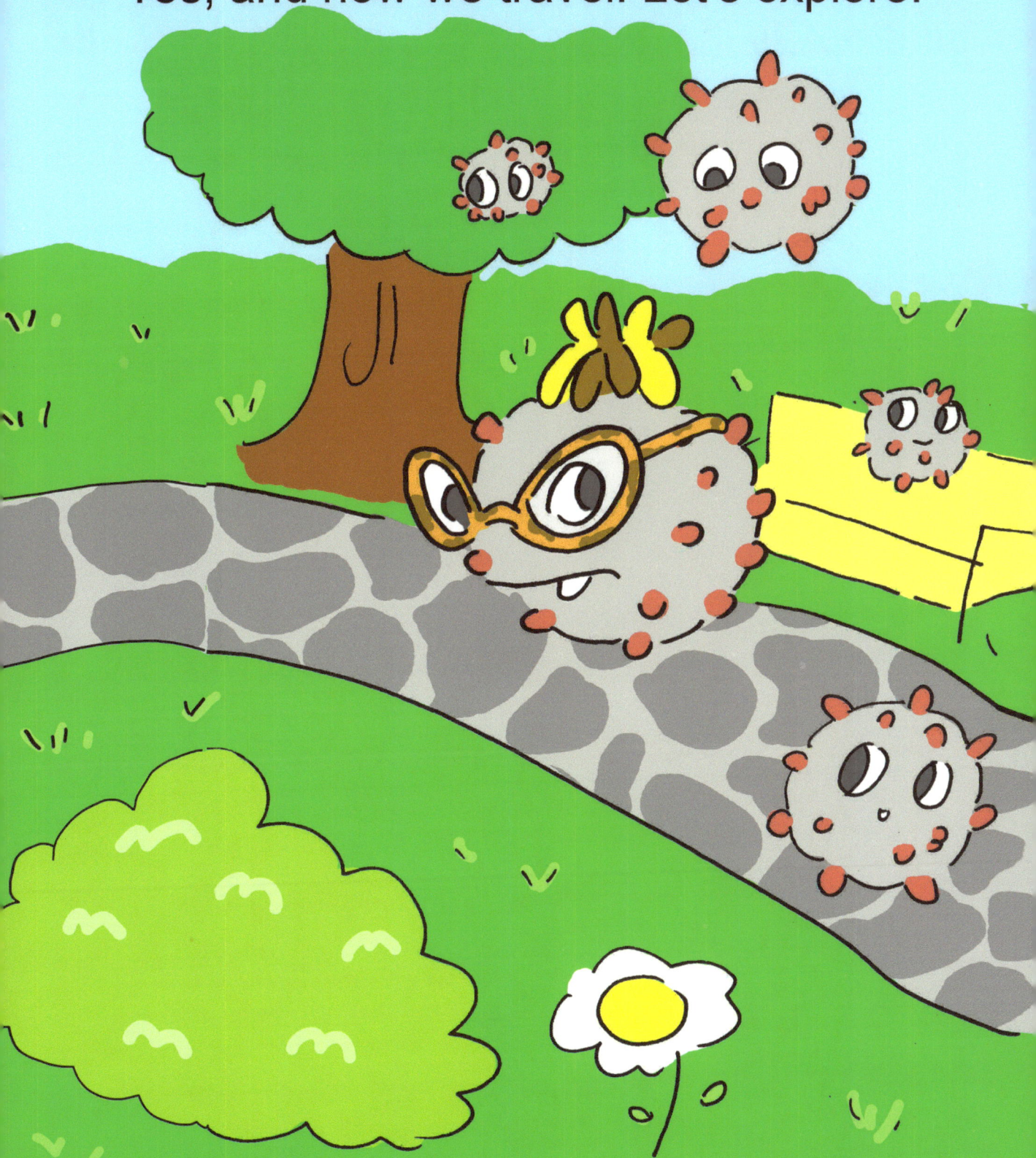

"Yes, and how we travel! Let's explore."

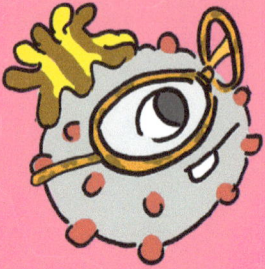

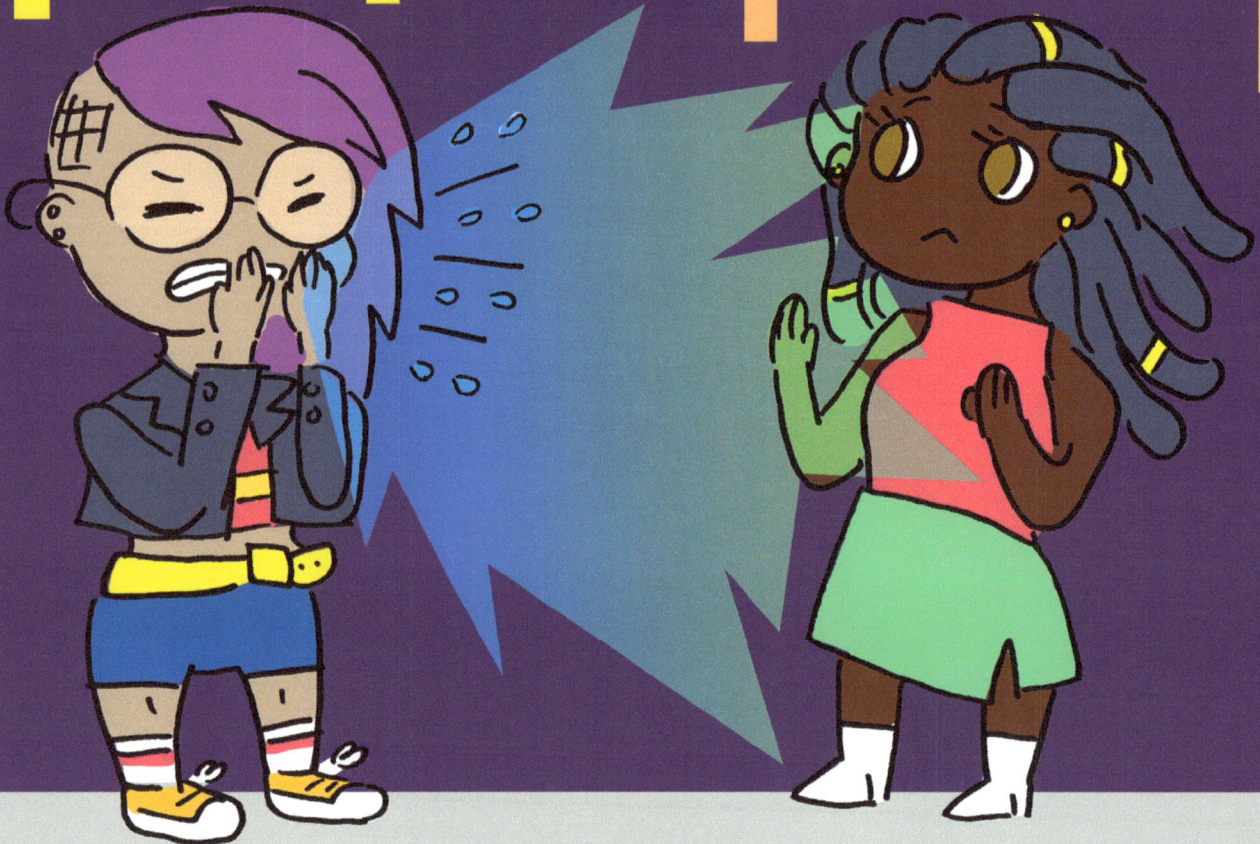

"This can happen with several diseases. And when we get into their bodies, they can get sick."

"They can have a cough, fever, and even trouble with breathing."

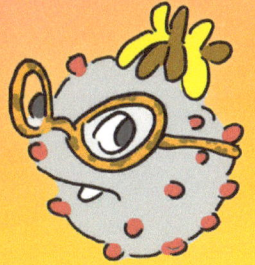

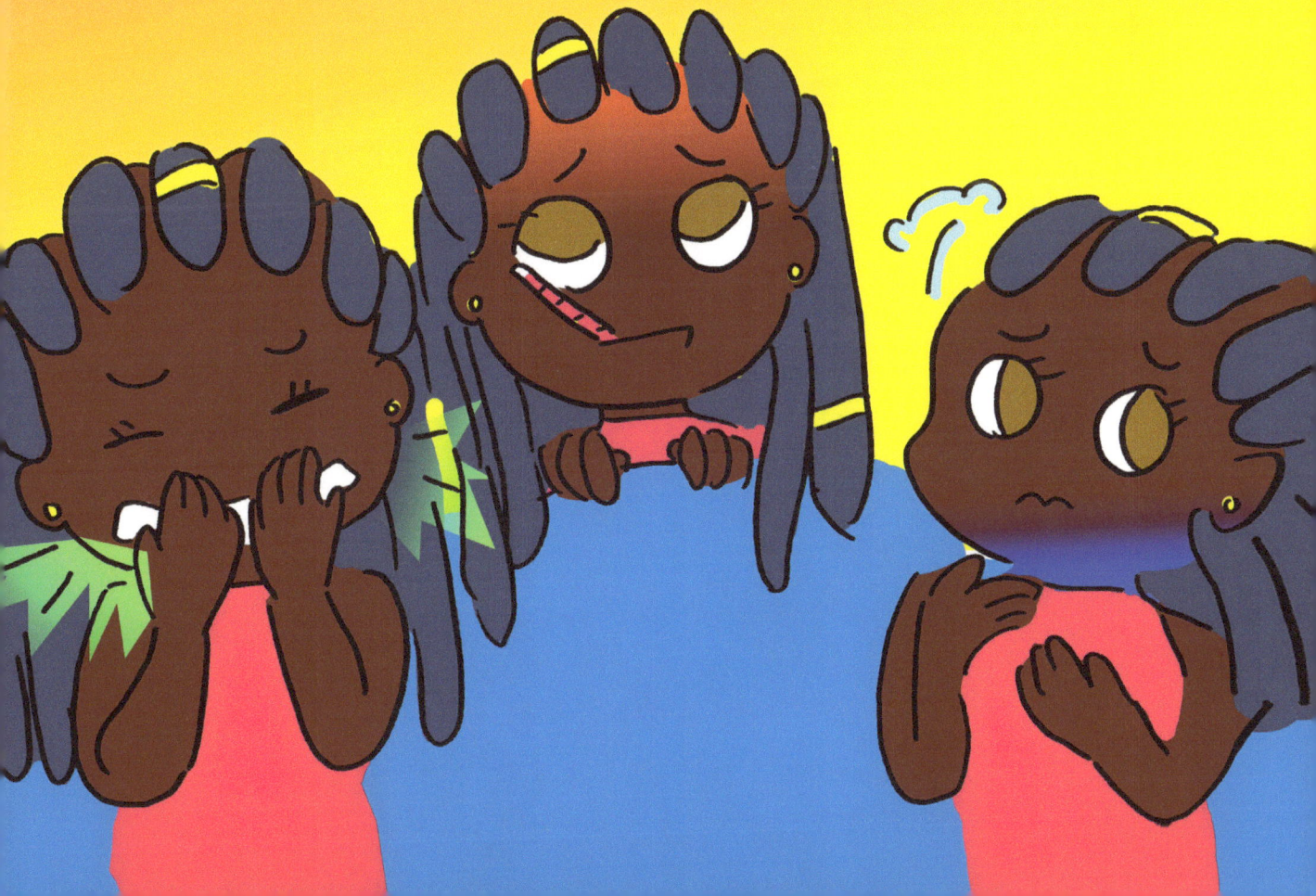

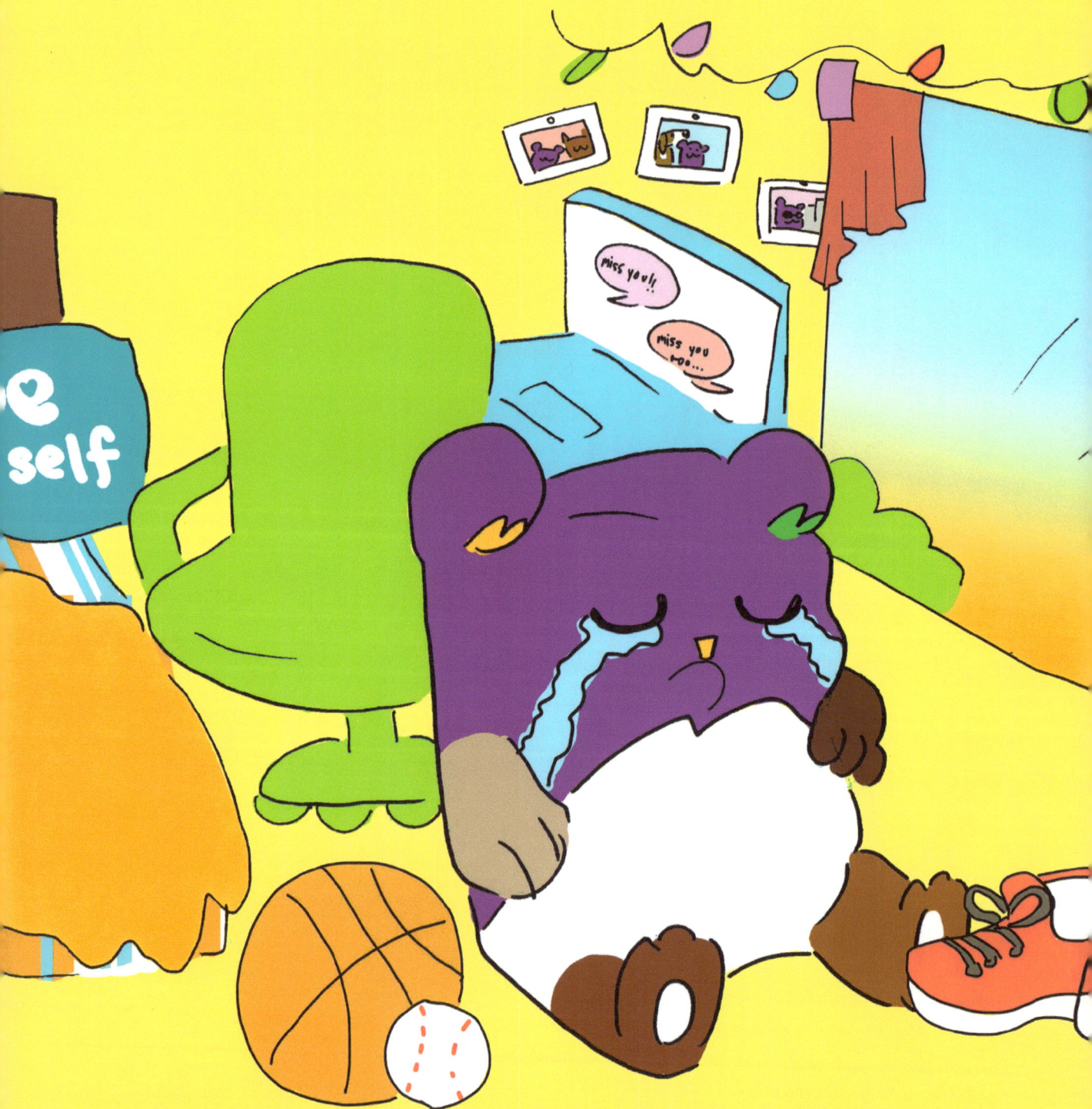

"Wow! Really? This makes me sad.
I feel like screaming!"

"It's okay to feel upset, Tickles.
Please know there are many people helping
to put a stop to this and keep you safe."

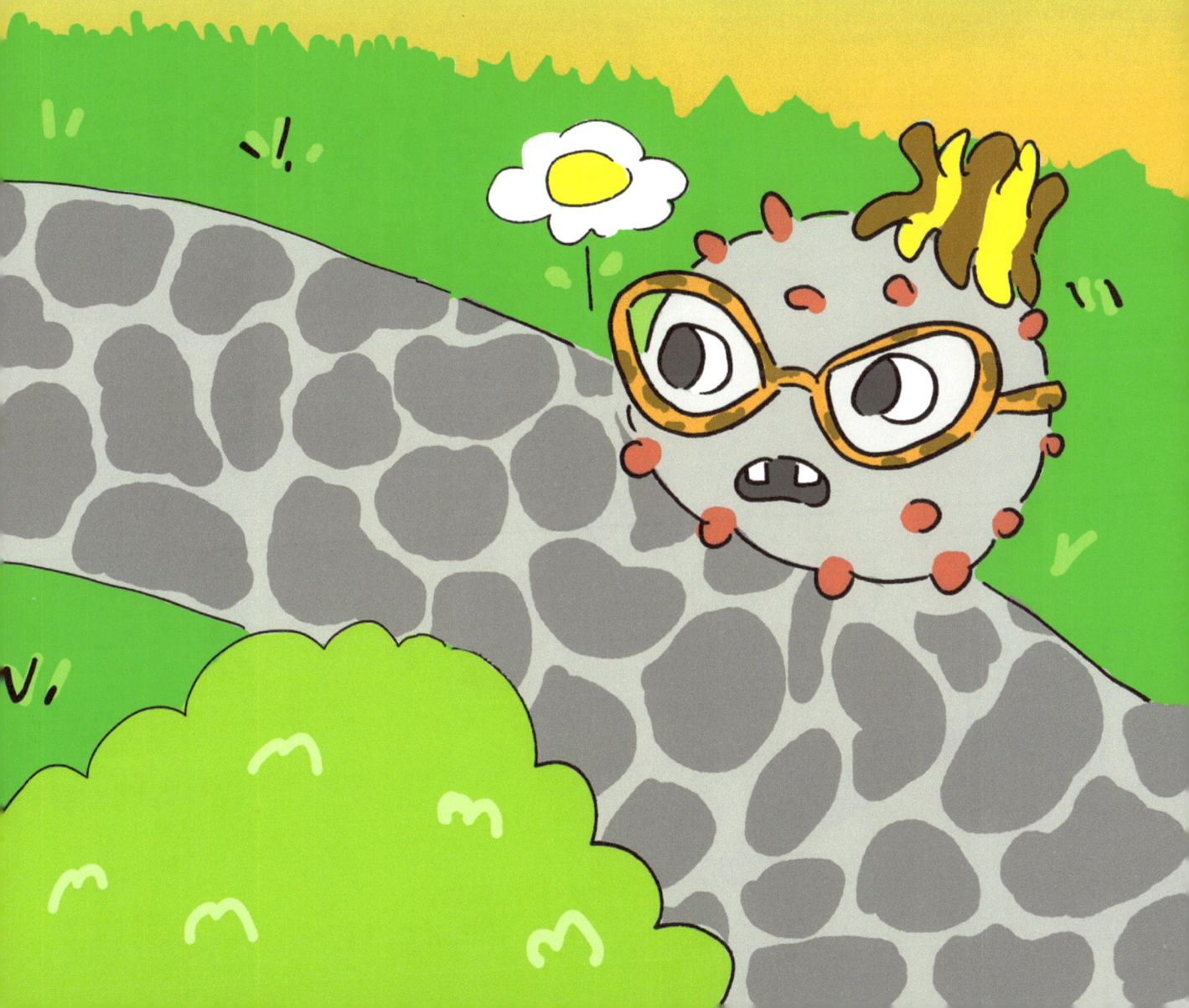

"Who are they?
Like me, they must be brave!"

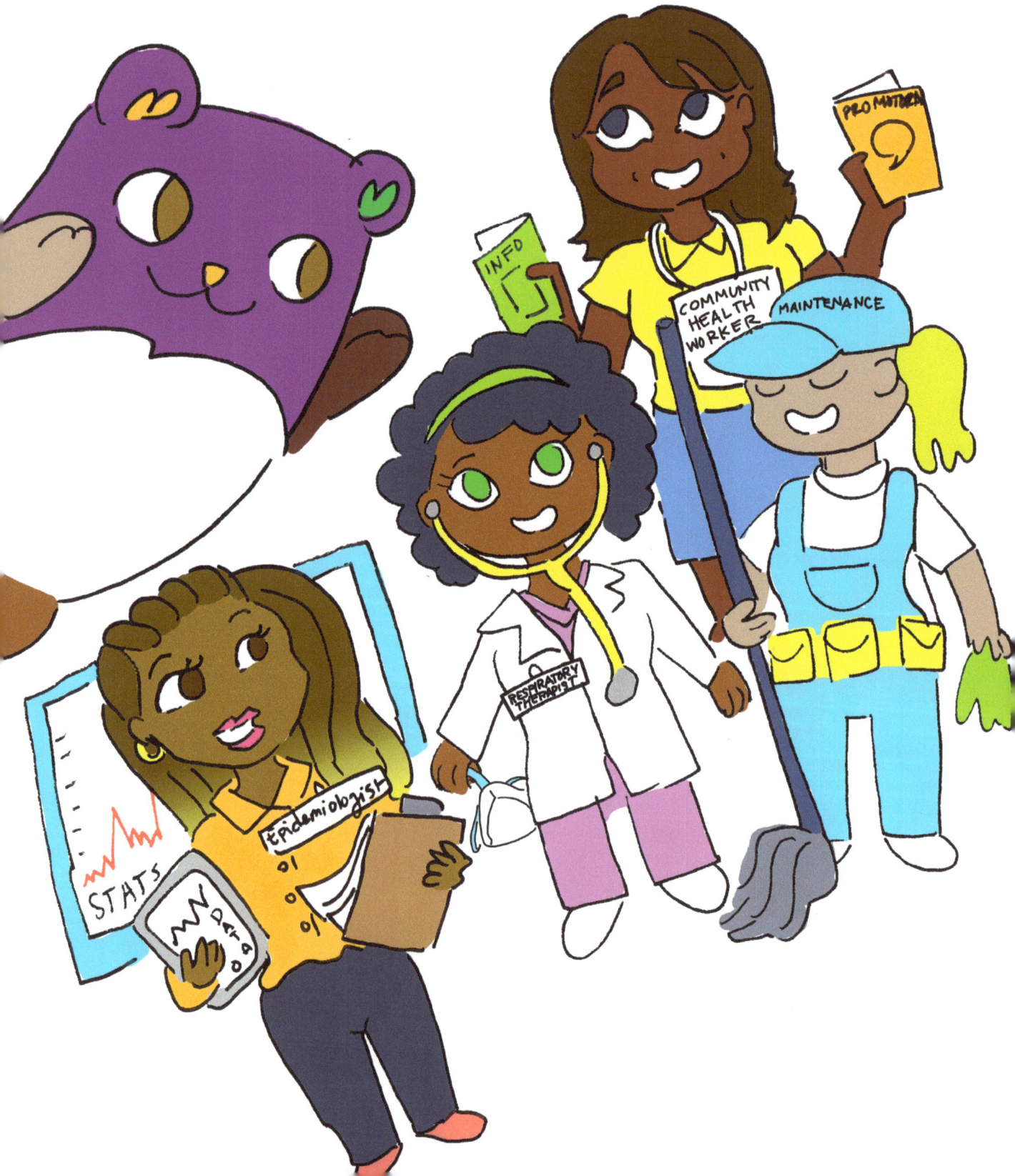

"You are right, Tickles.
And every day,
because of their helping hands,
we may stay safe."

"They are world leaders, scientists,
all kinds of health care workers
and public health staff."

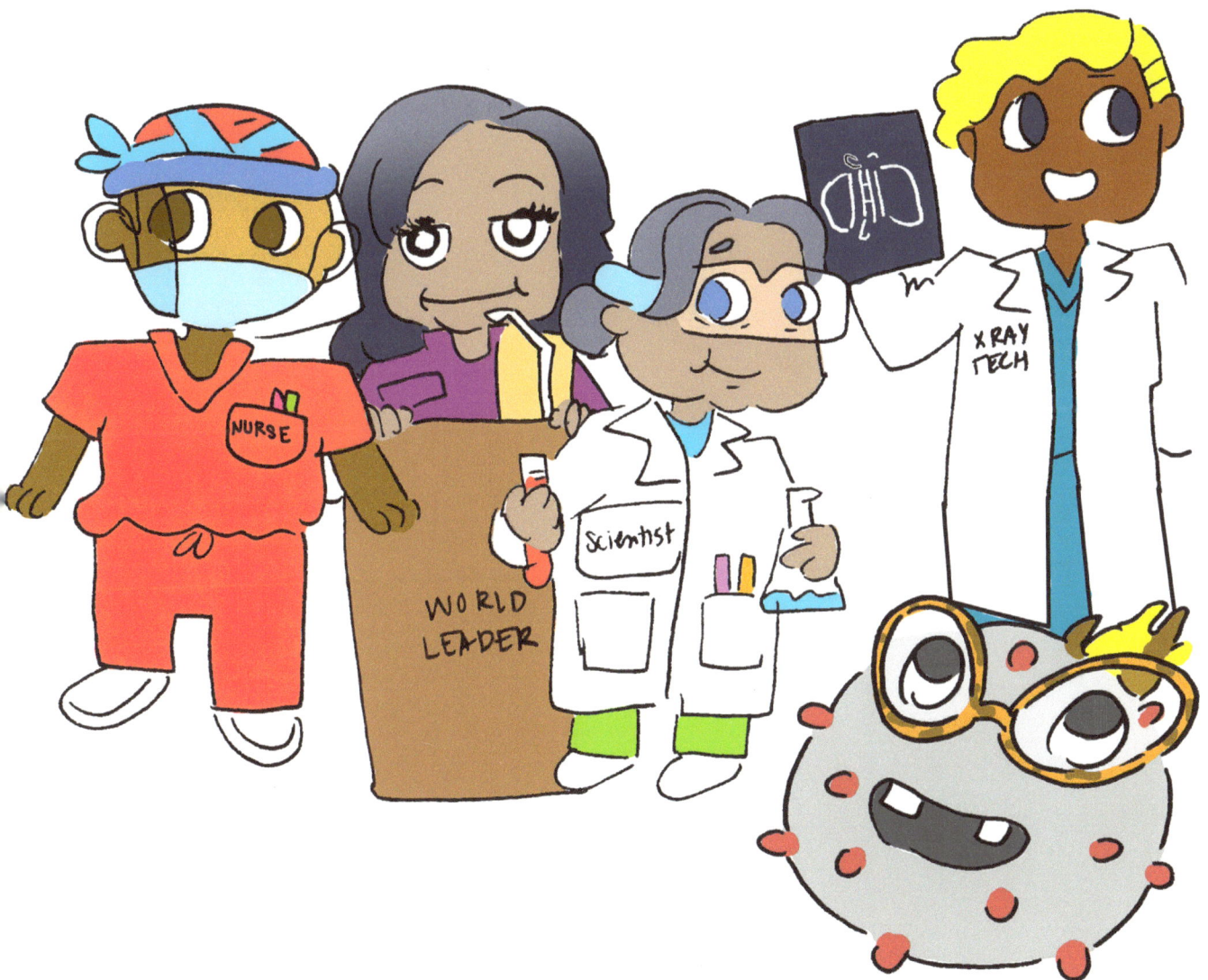

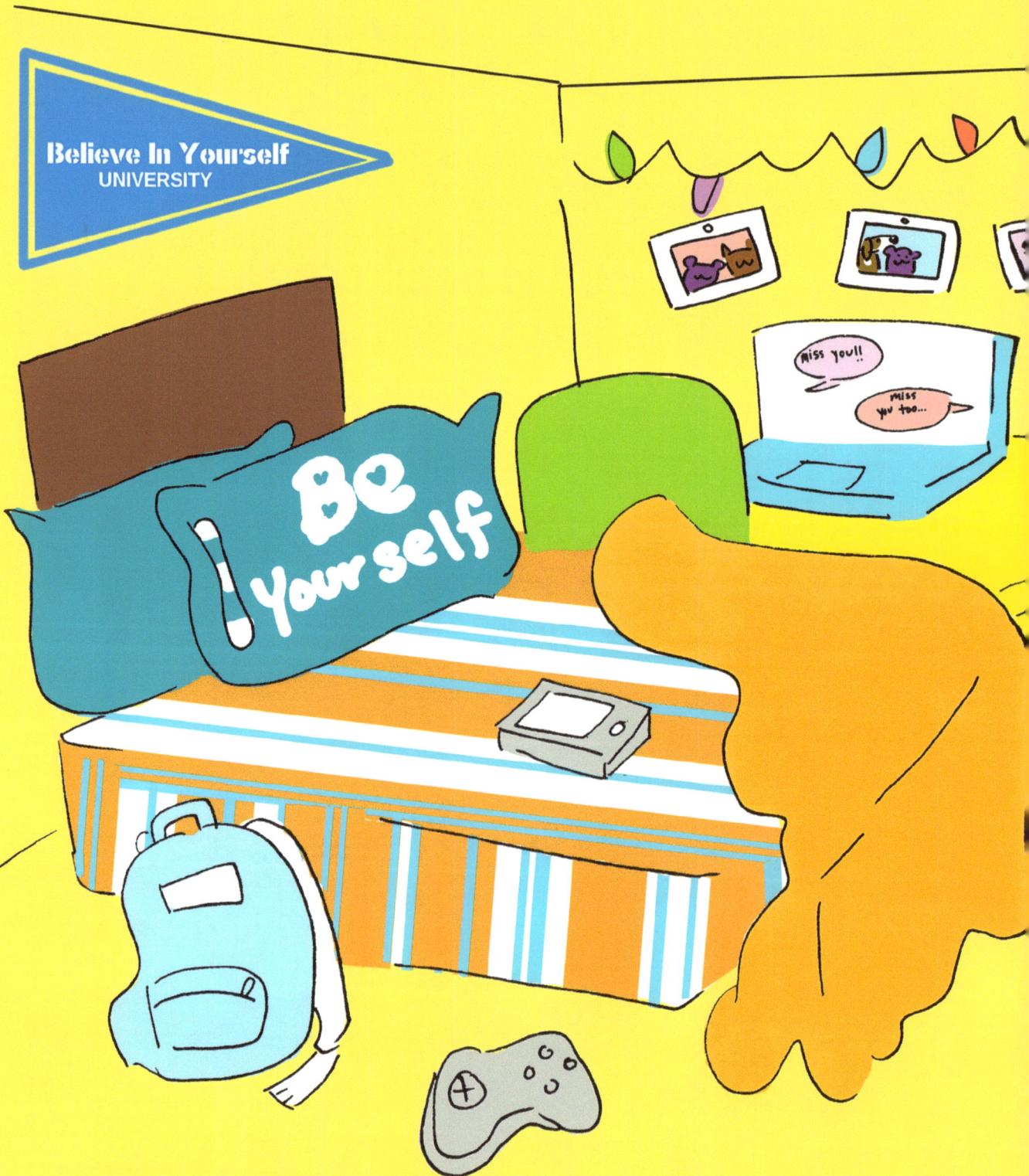
"This makes me happy again! I can just laugh."

"And that's not all. That's only half."

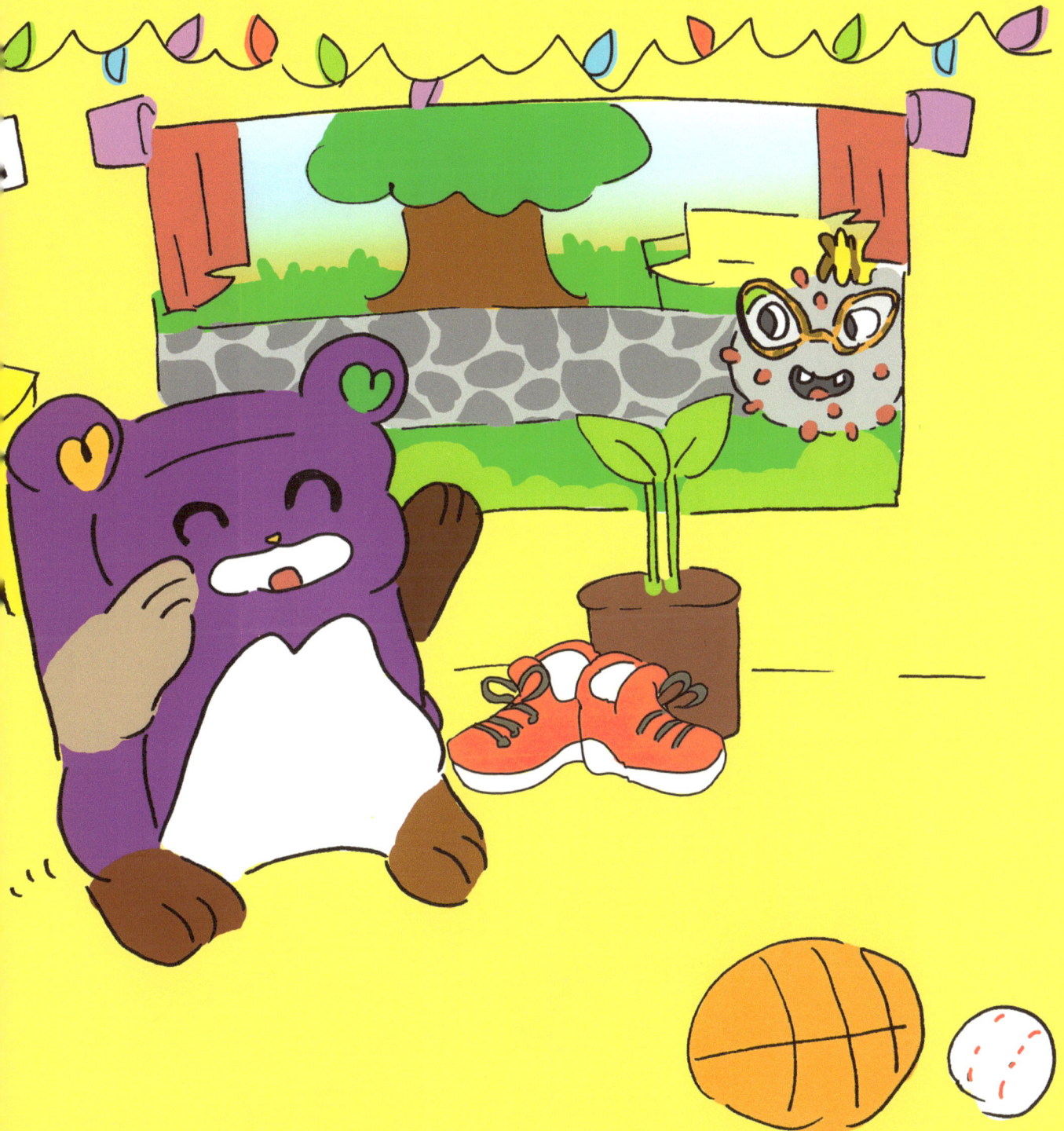

"Many others are helping too.
Some are community helpers, bus and
truck drivers, store and restaurant workers,
and workers in schools."

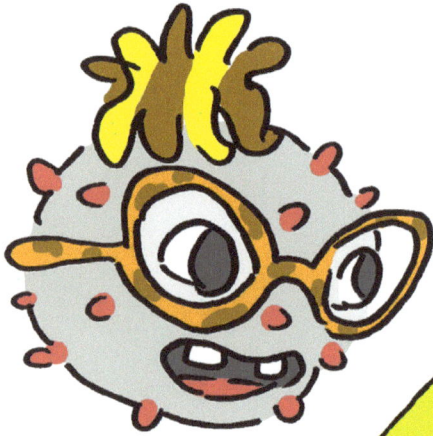

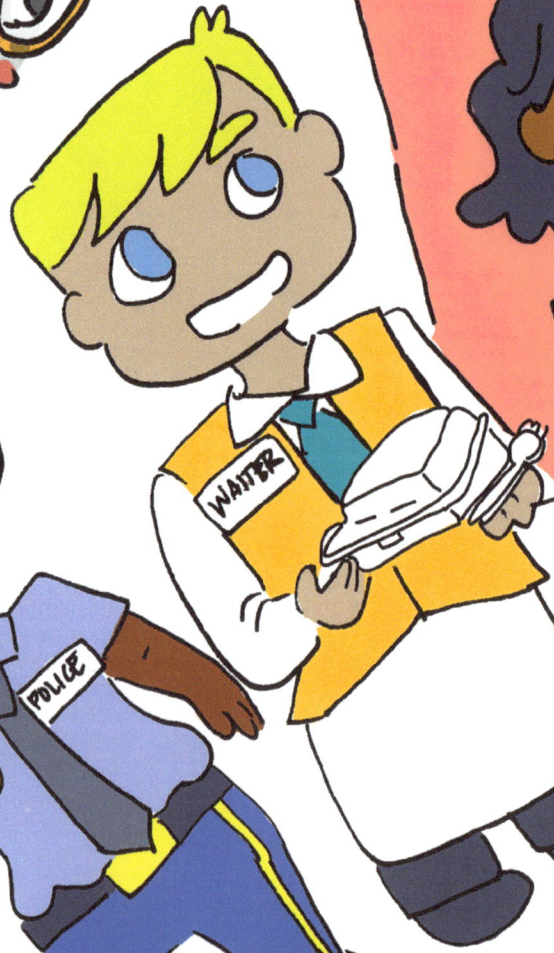

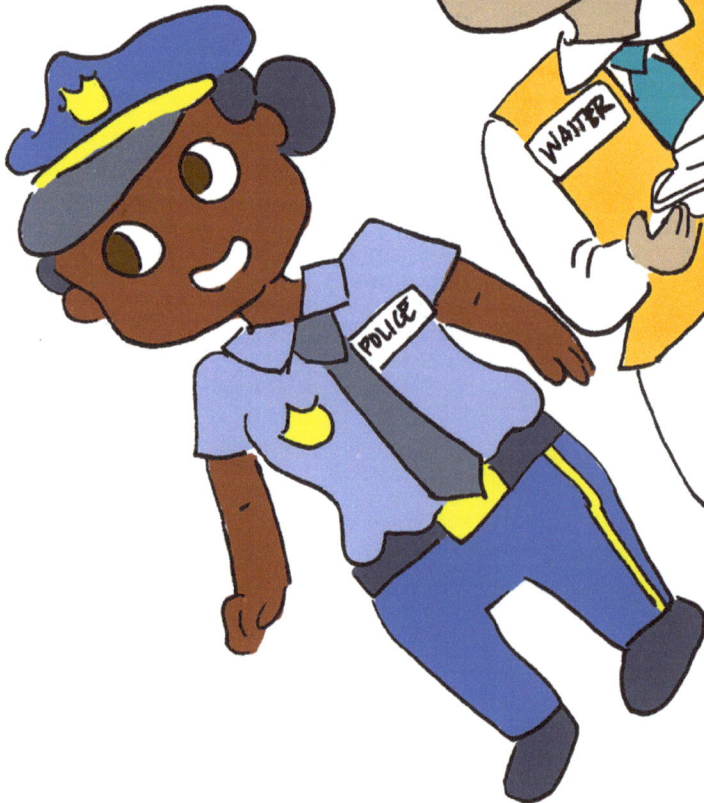

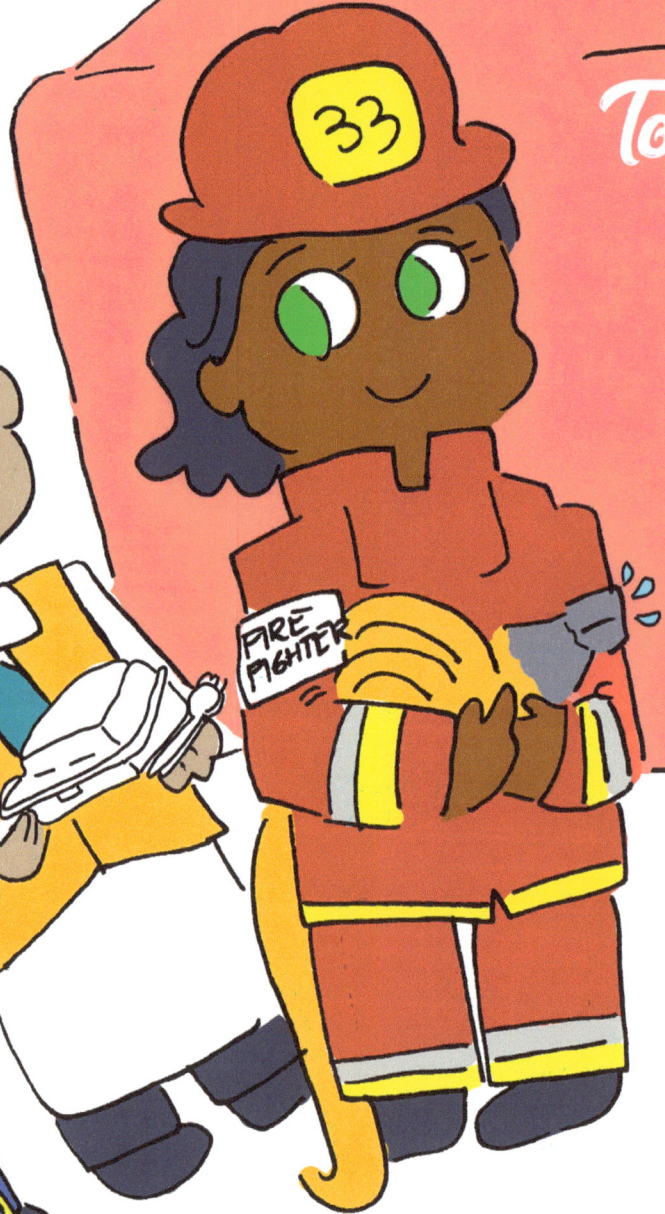

"They are all great!
This is so cool."

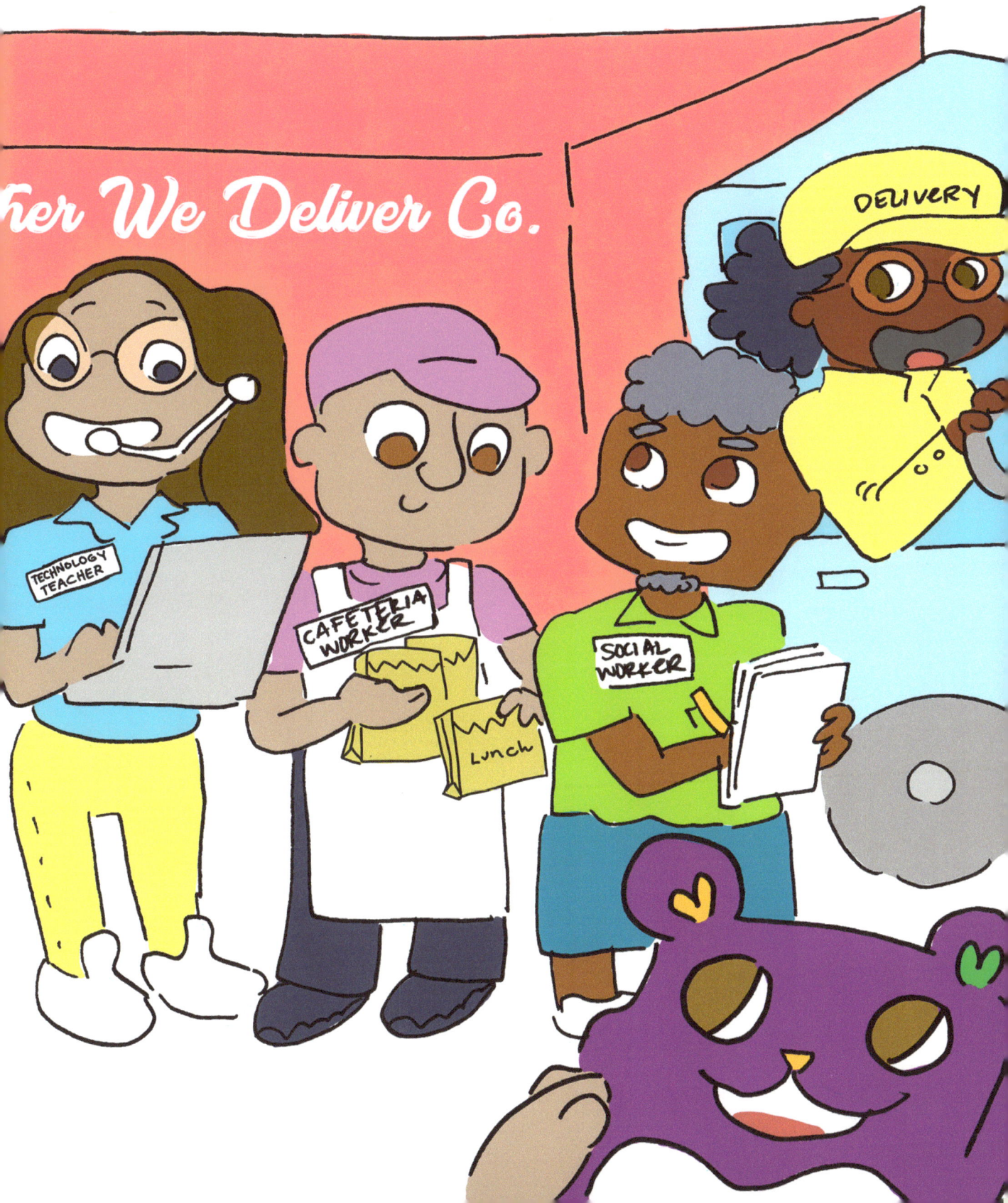

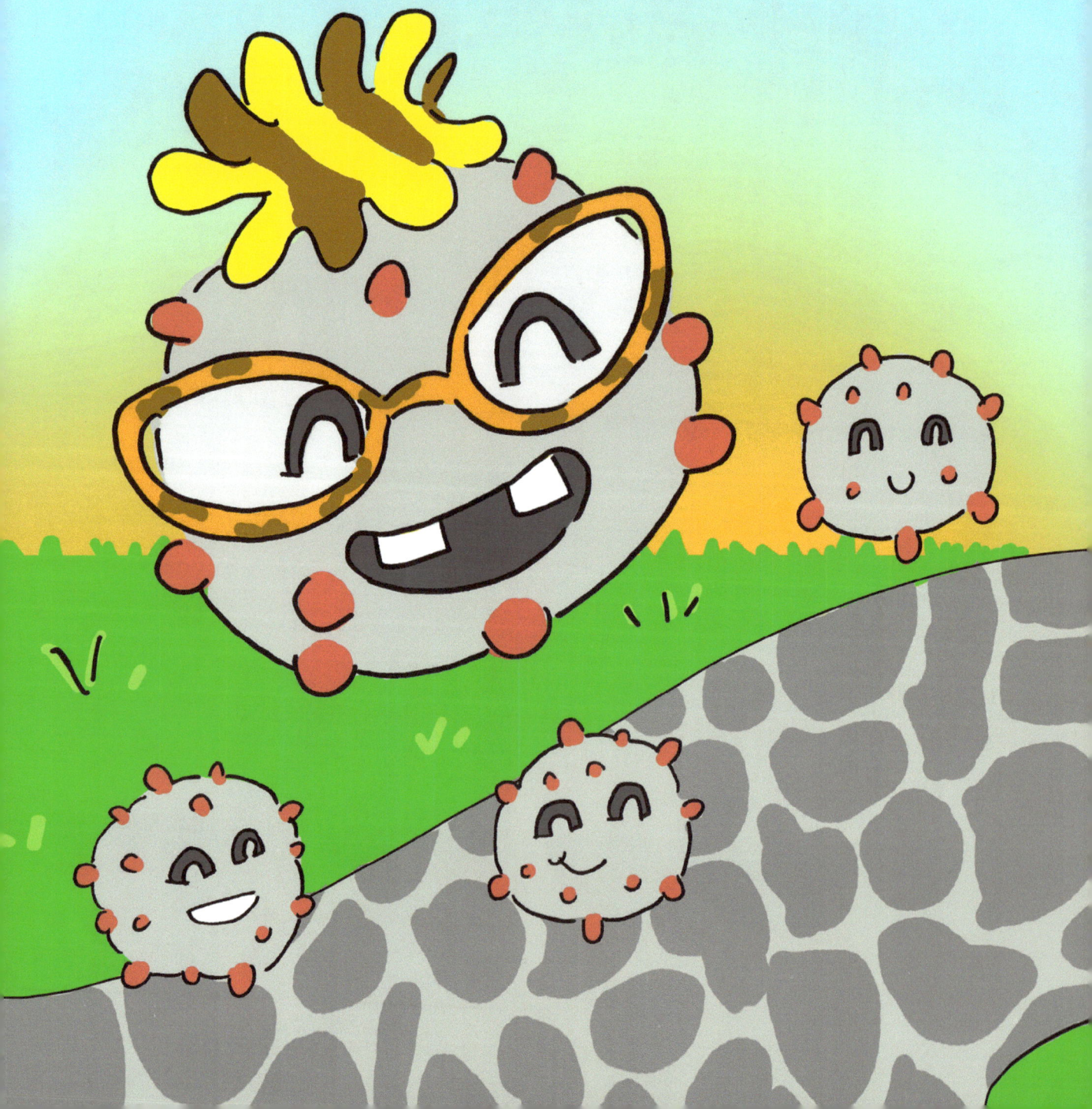

"Yes! And there are things you and your family can do to help too."

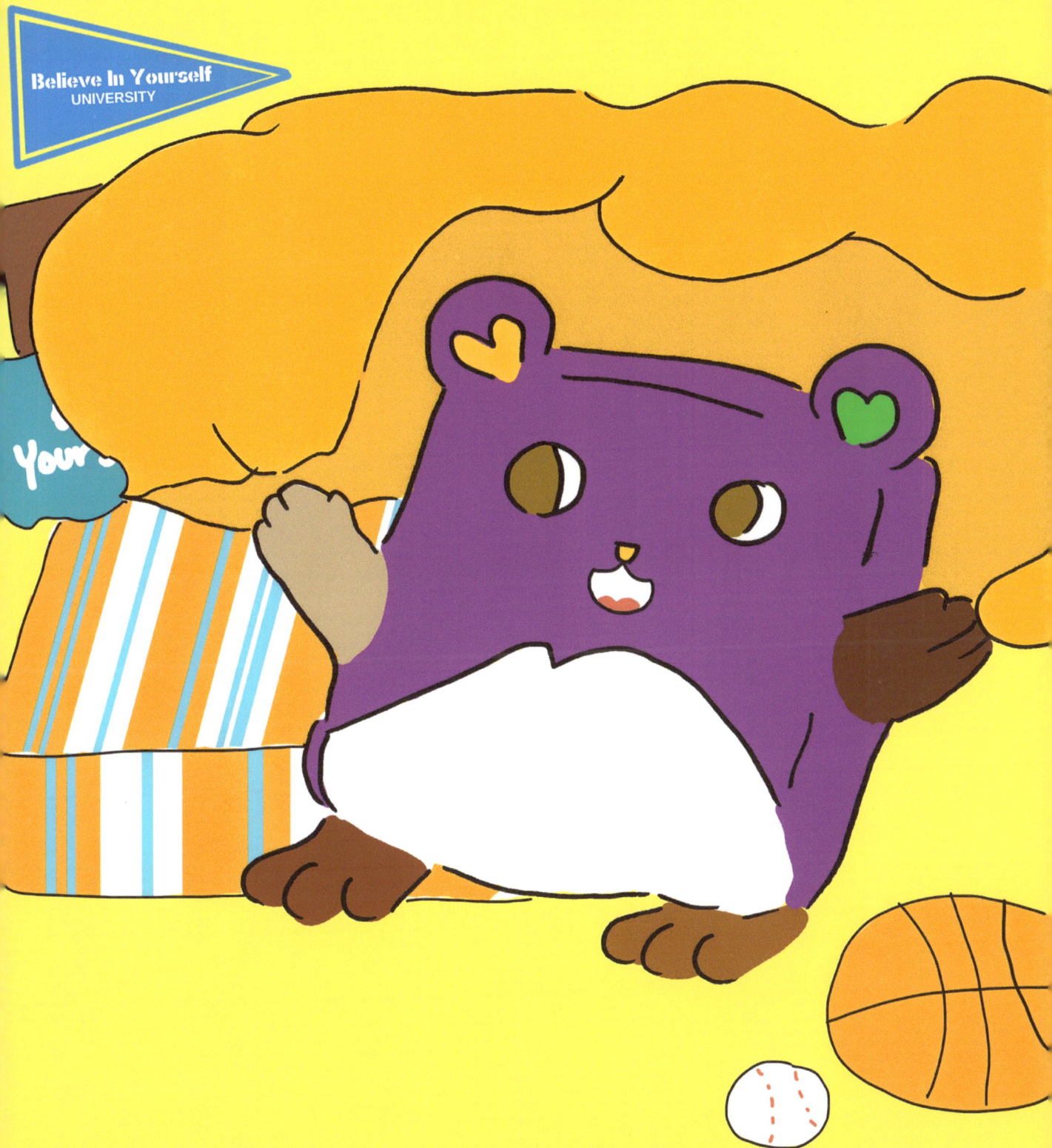

"You can wash your hands for
at least 20 seconds each time."

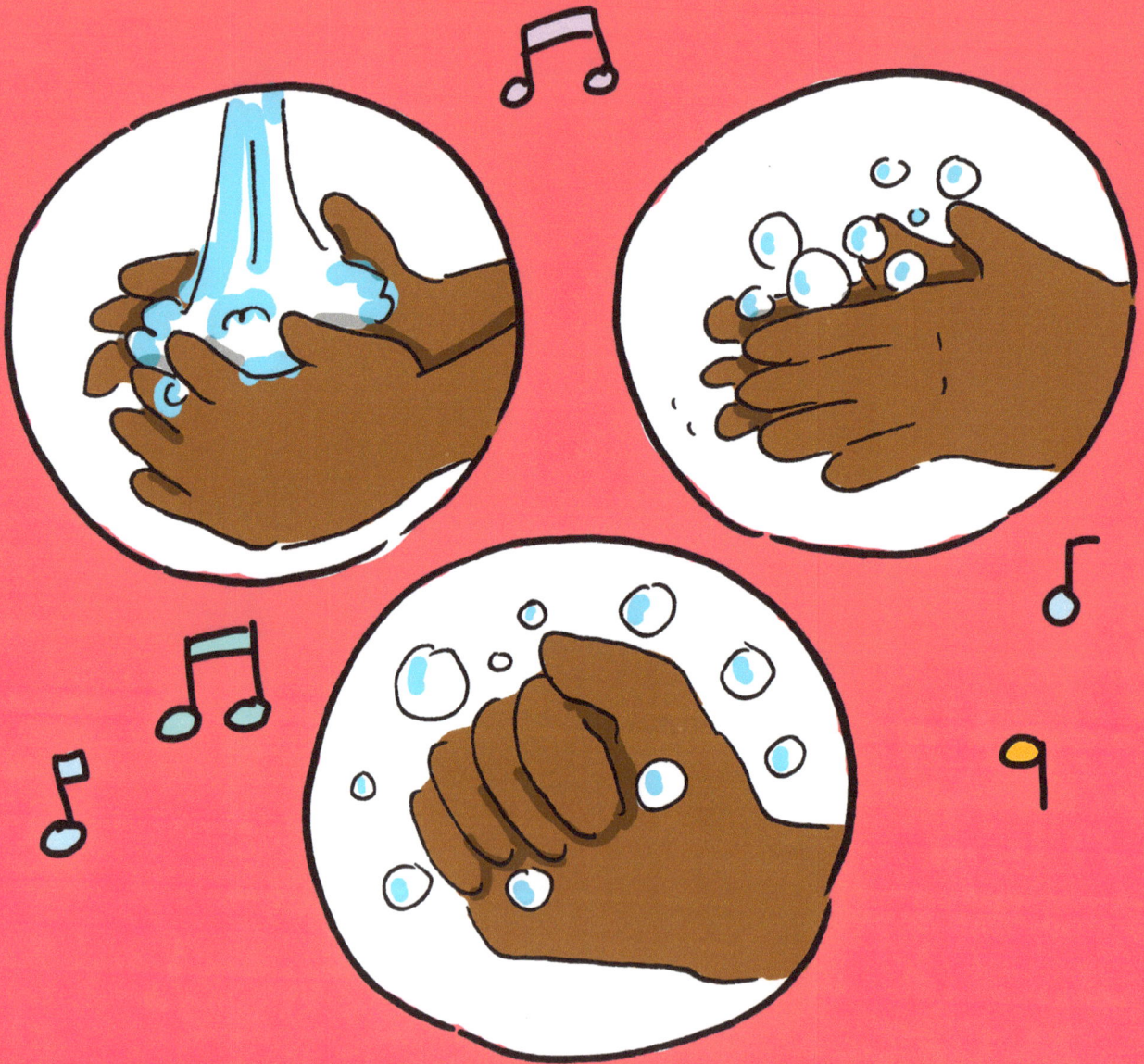

"If you do it while singing
the 'Happy Birthday' song twice,
this can help make sure it's done right."

"I can do this, with all of my might!"

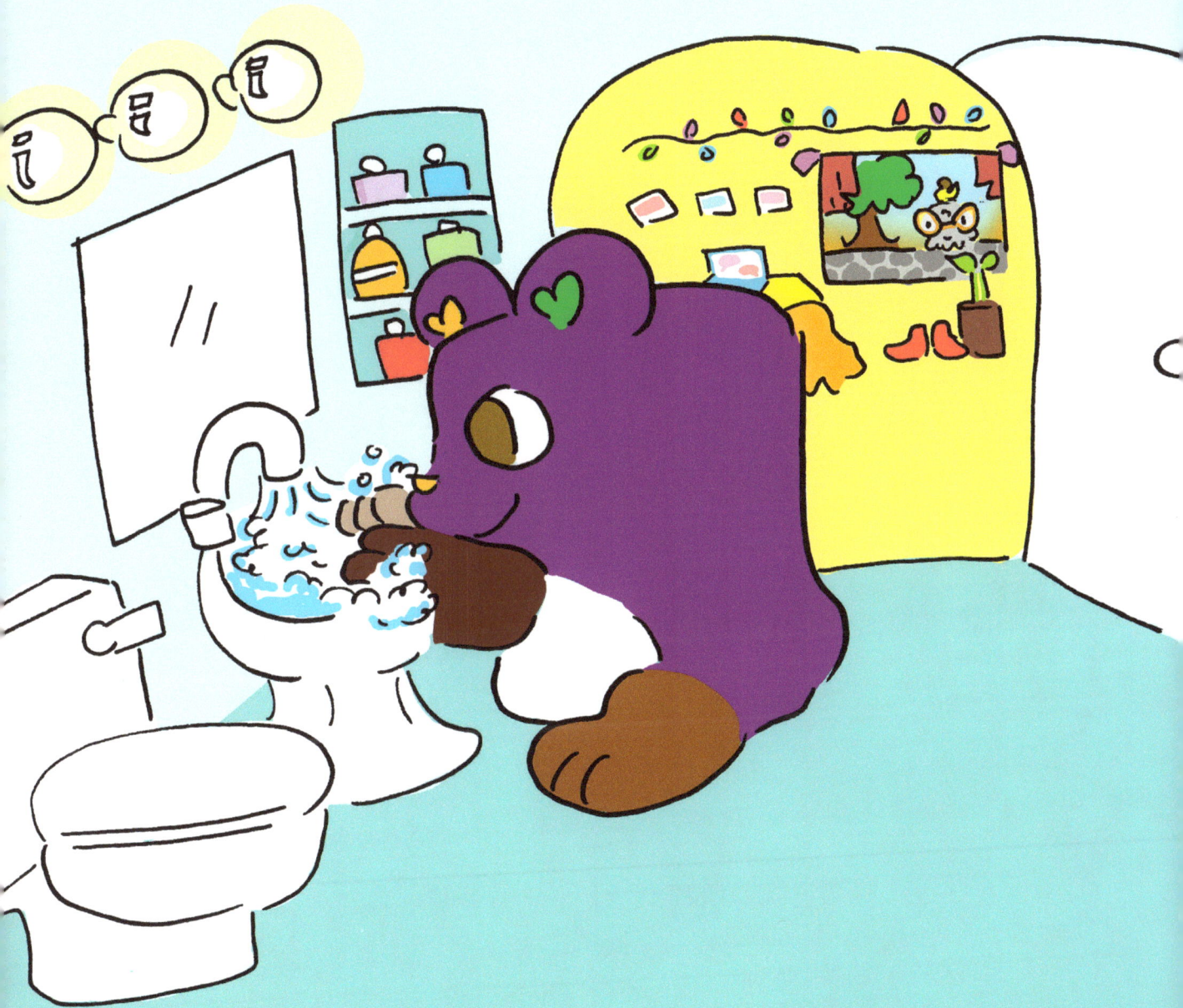

"You sure can, Tickles!
You and your family can also
use social distancing when going to places
like the grocery store or park."

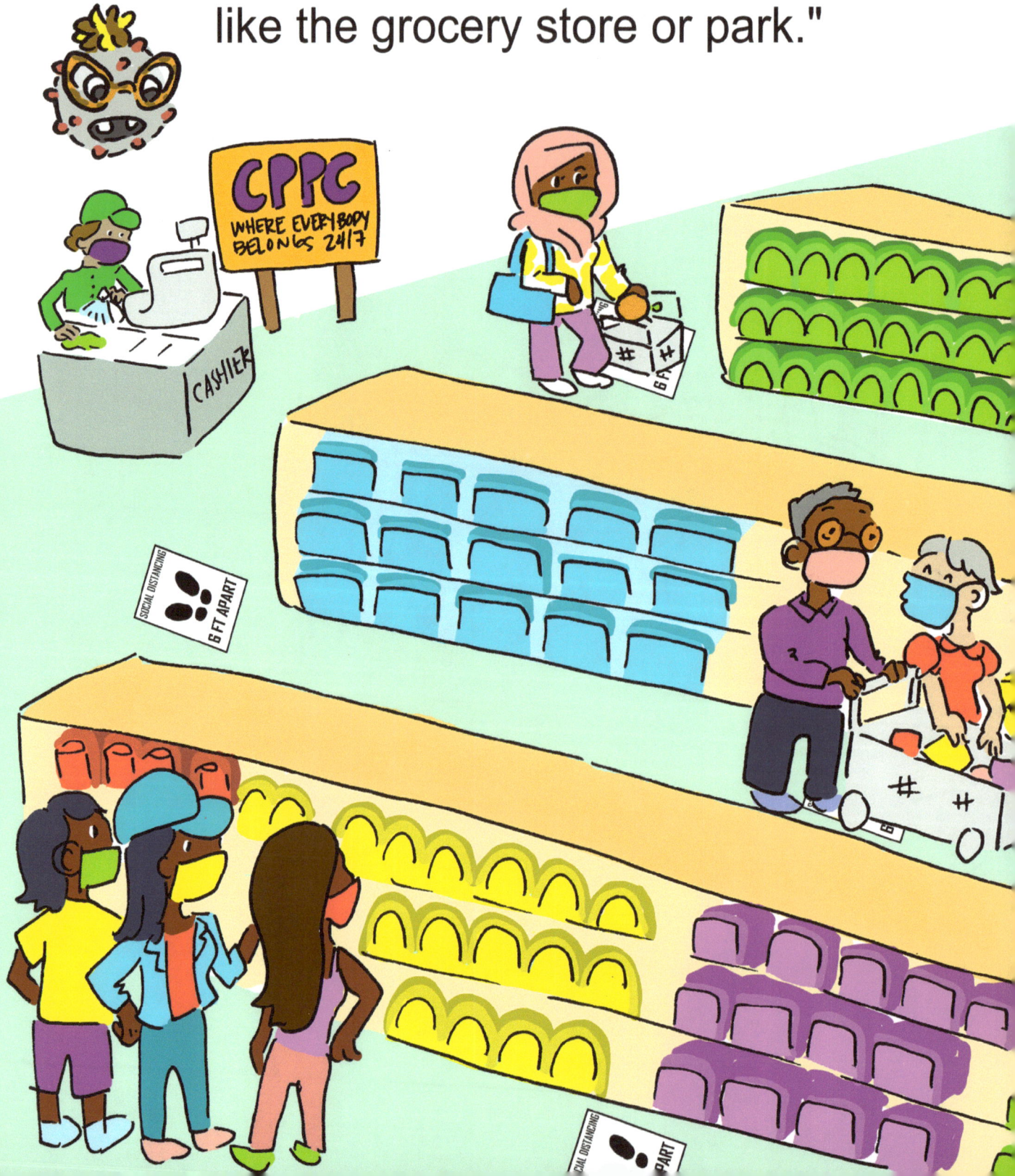

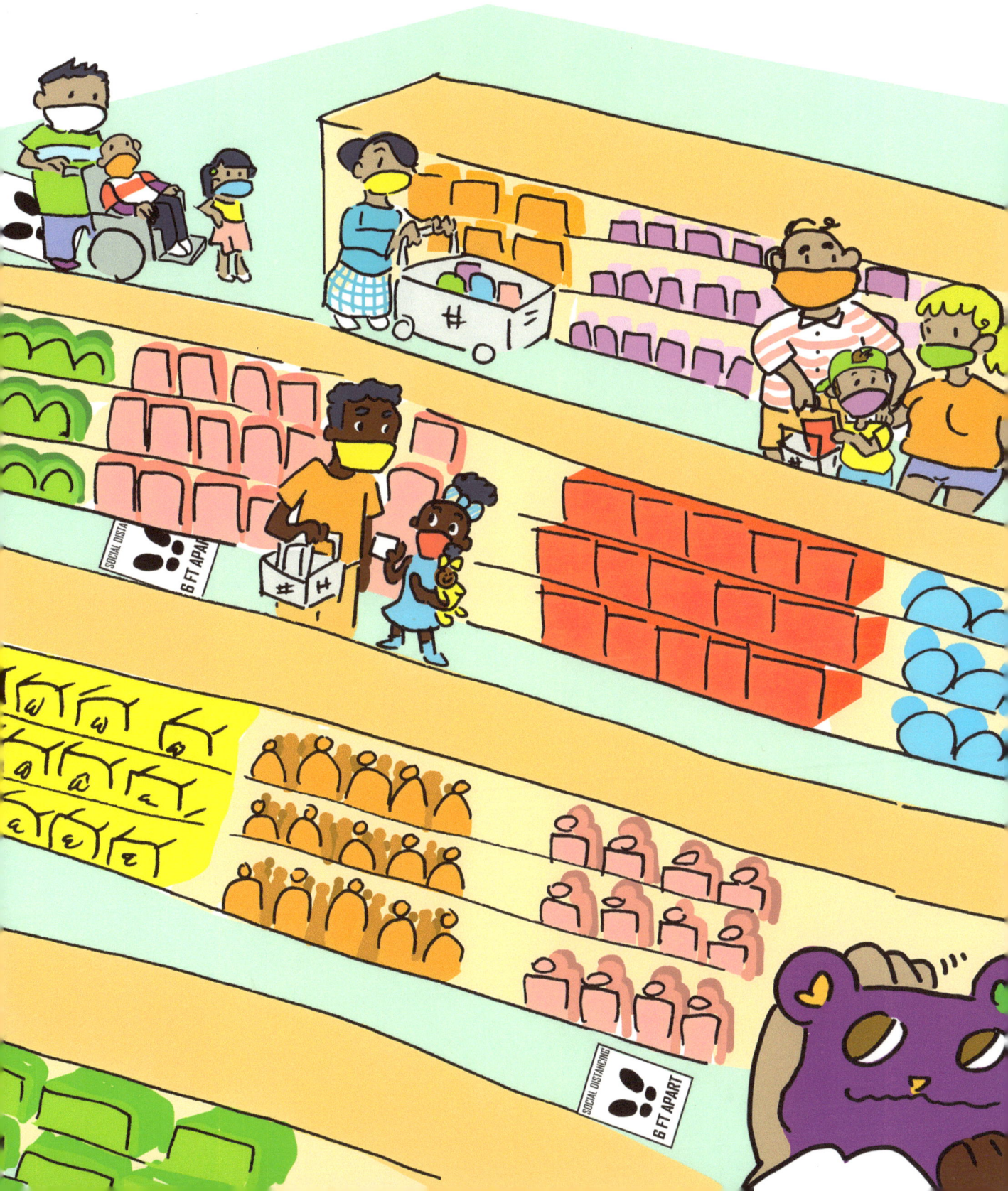

"Sooocio…what?
Can you please restart?"

"Social distancing is when you stand or sit at least 6 feet apart."

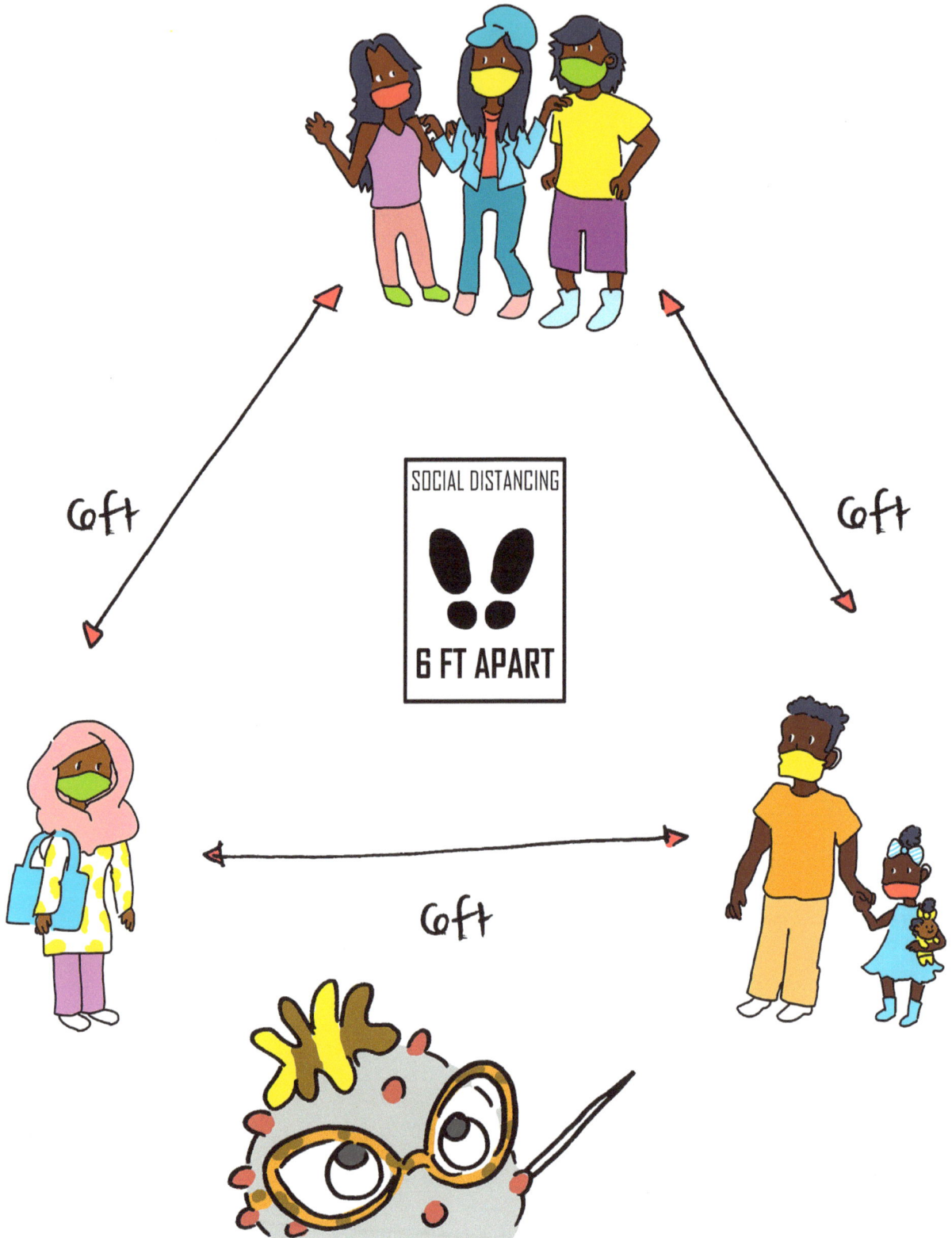

SOCIAL DISTANCING

6 FT APART

6ft

6ft

6ft

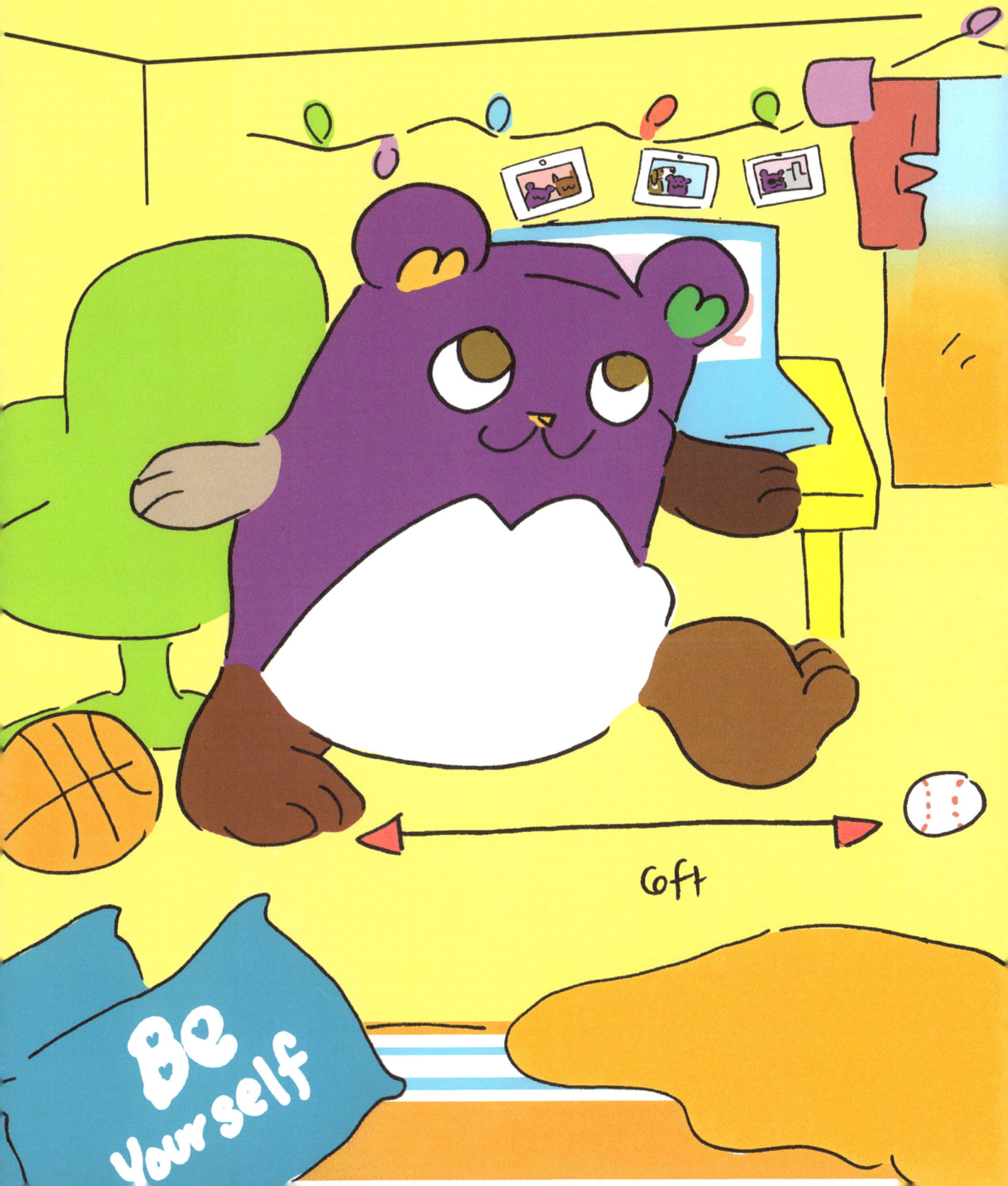
"Hmmm…I think that would look something like 6 big steps on a foot chart."

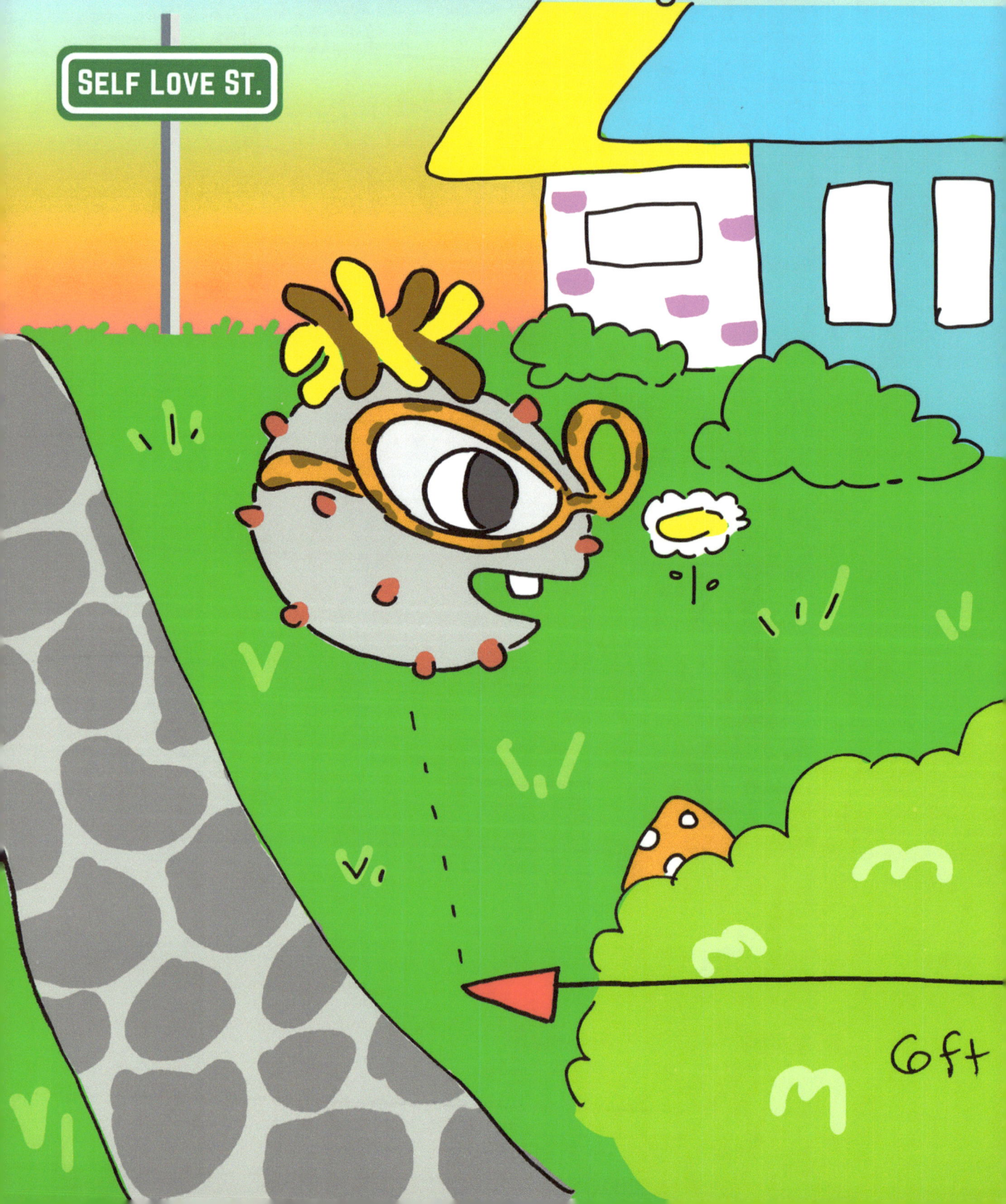

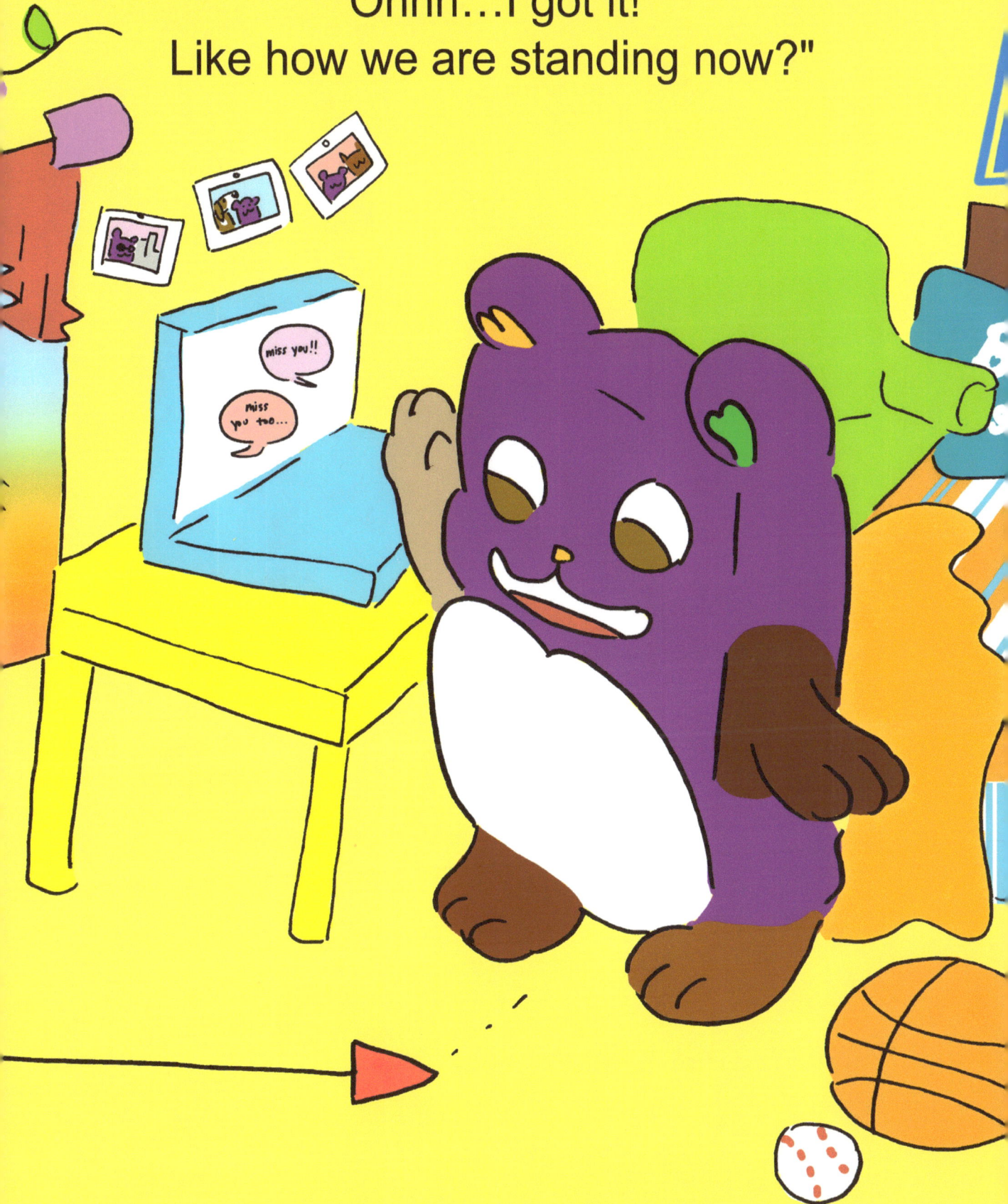

"Ohhh…I got it!
Like how we are standing now?"

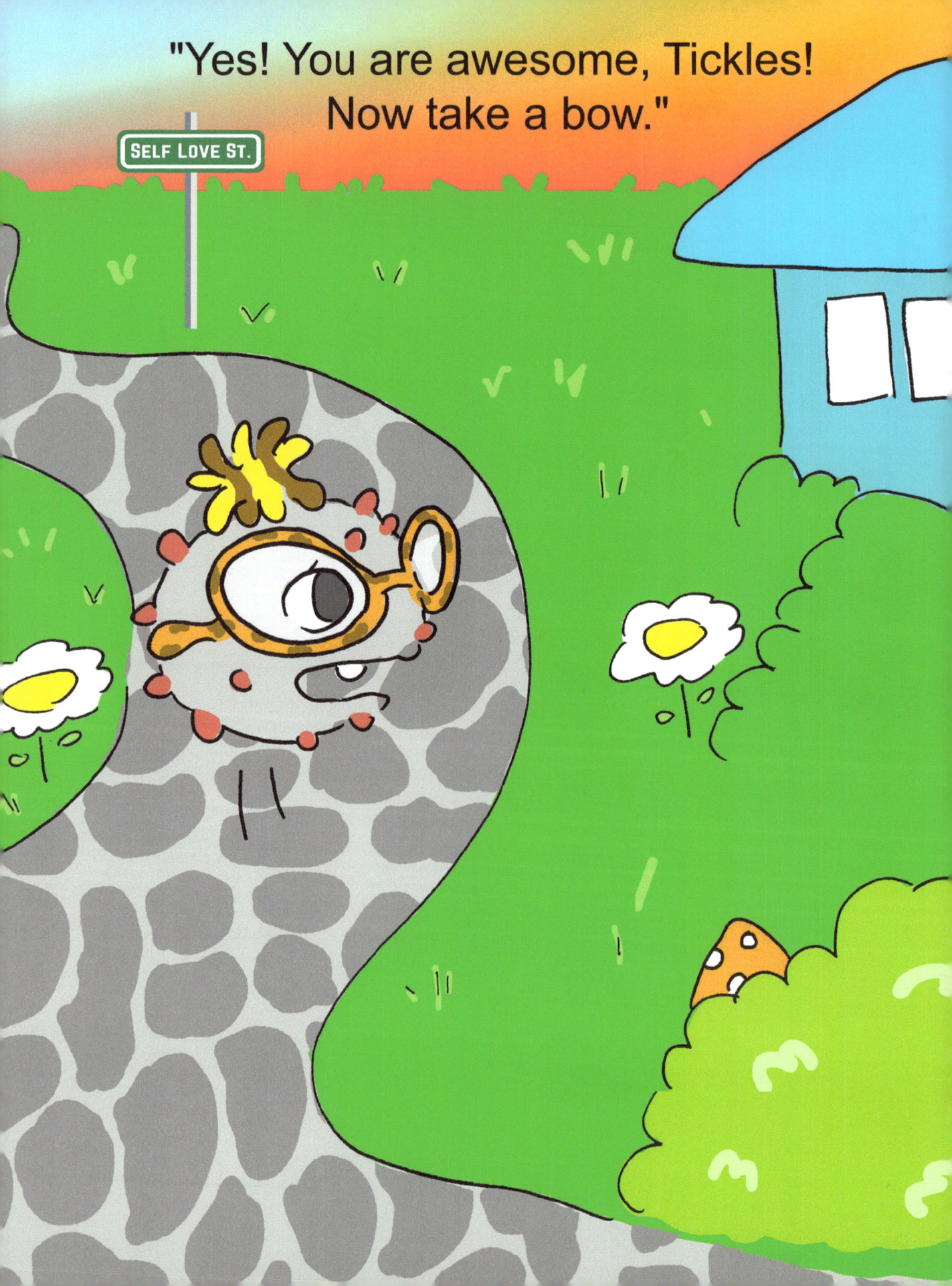

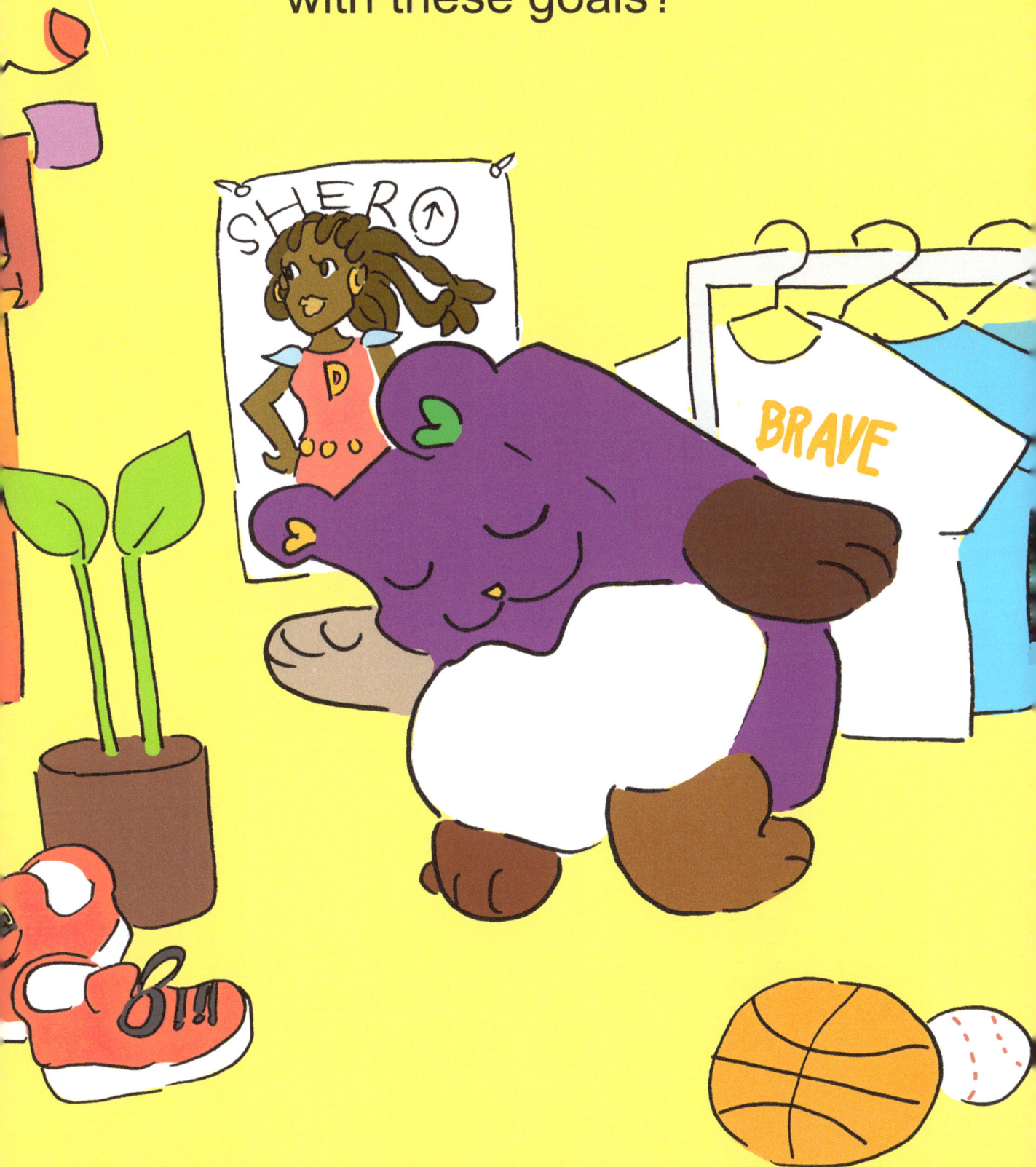

"Pow! I am on a roll.
What else can we do to help
with these goals?"

"In your favorite bowl, you can enjoy fruits and vegetables to help keep your body healthy."

"And taking time for rest is a big deal too."

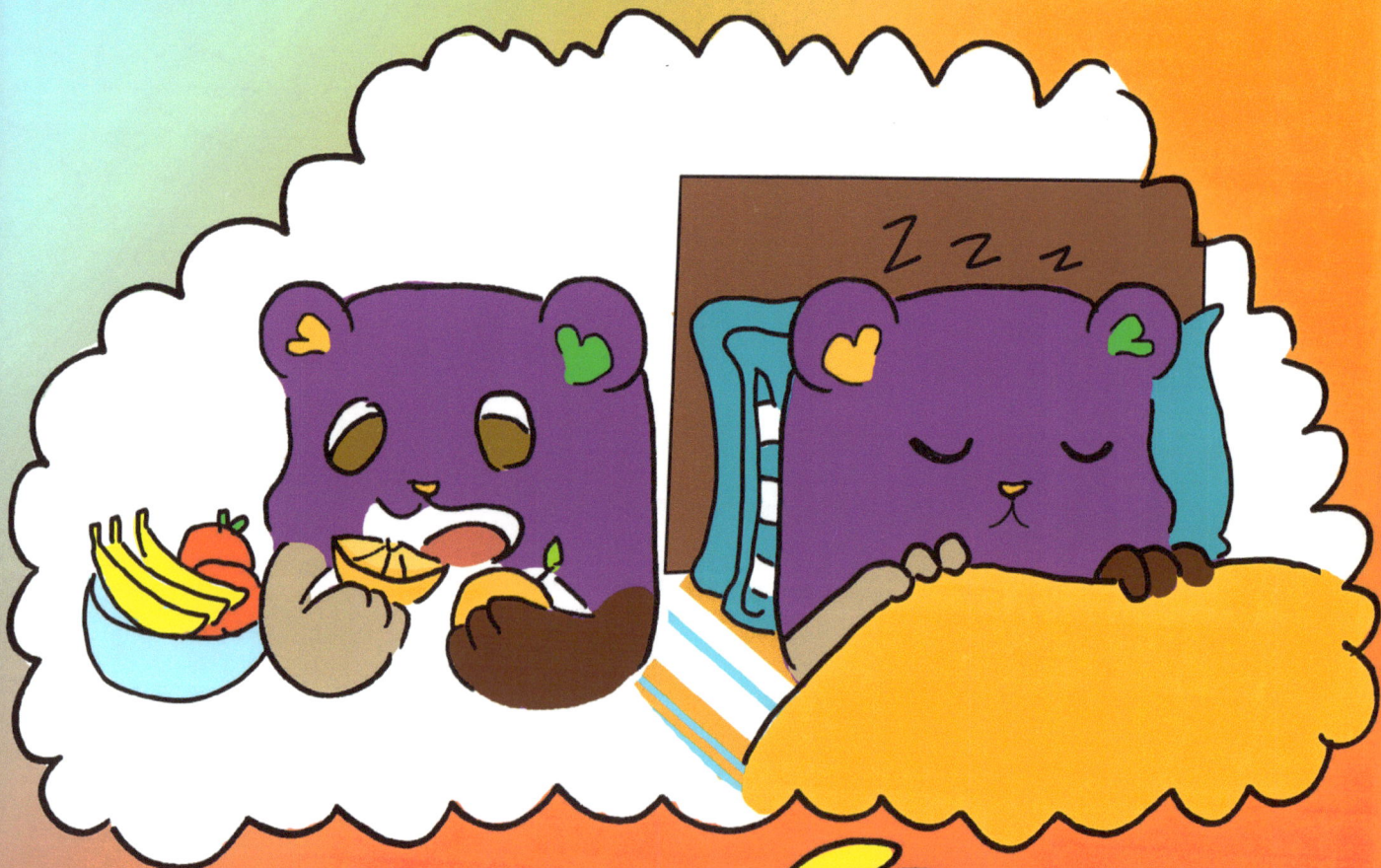

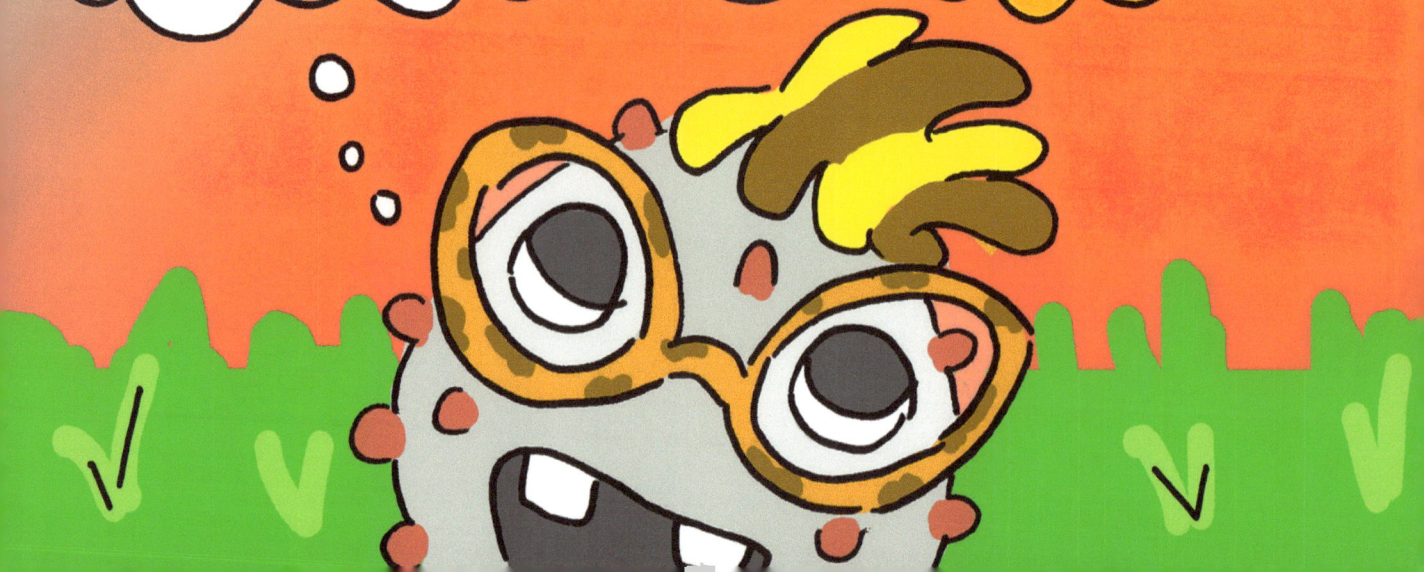

"This all sounds good.
But what if I'm sad again.
What do I do?"

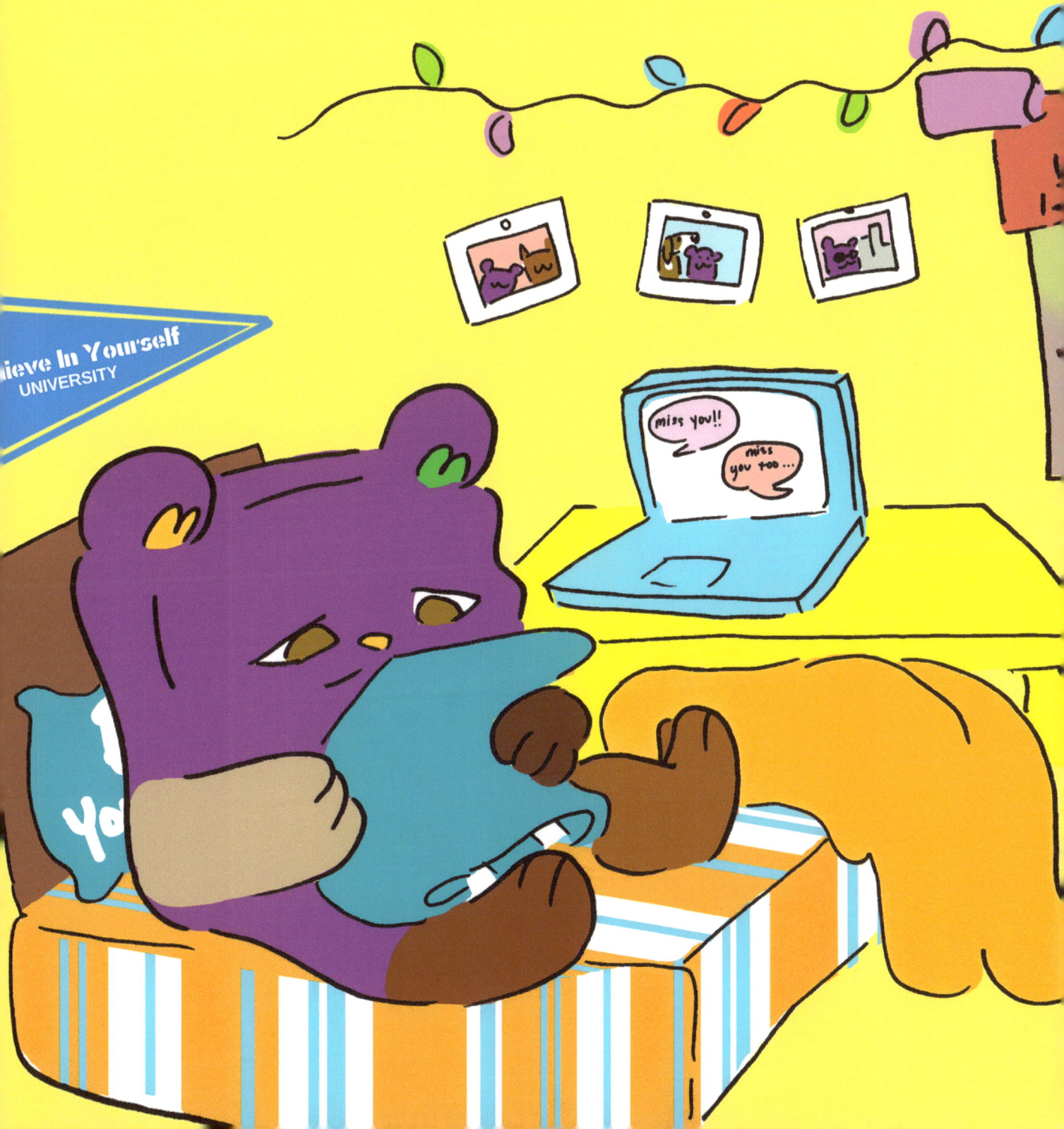

"You don't have to lose hope.
You can talk to an adult about your feelings,
and write in a journal to help you cope."

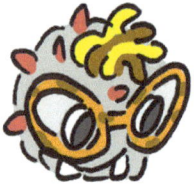

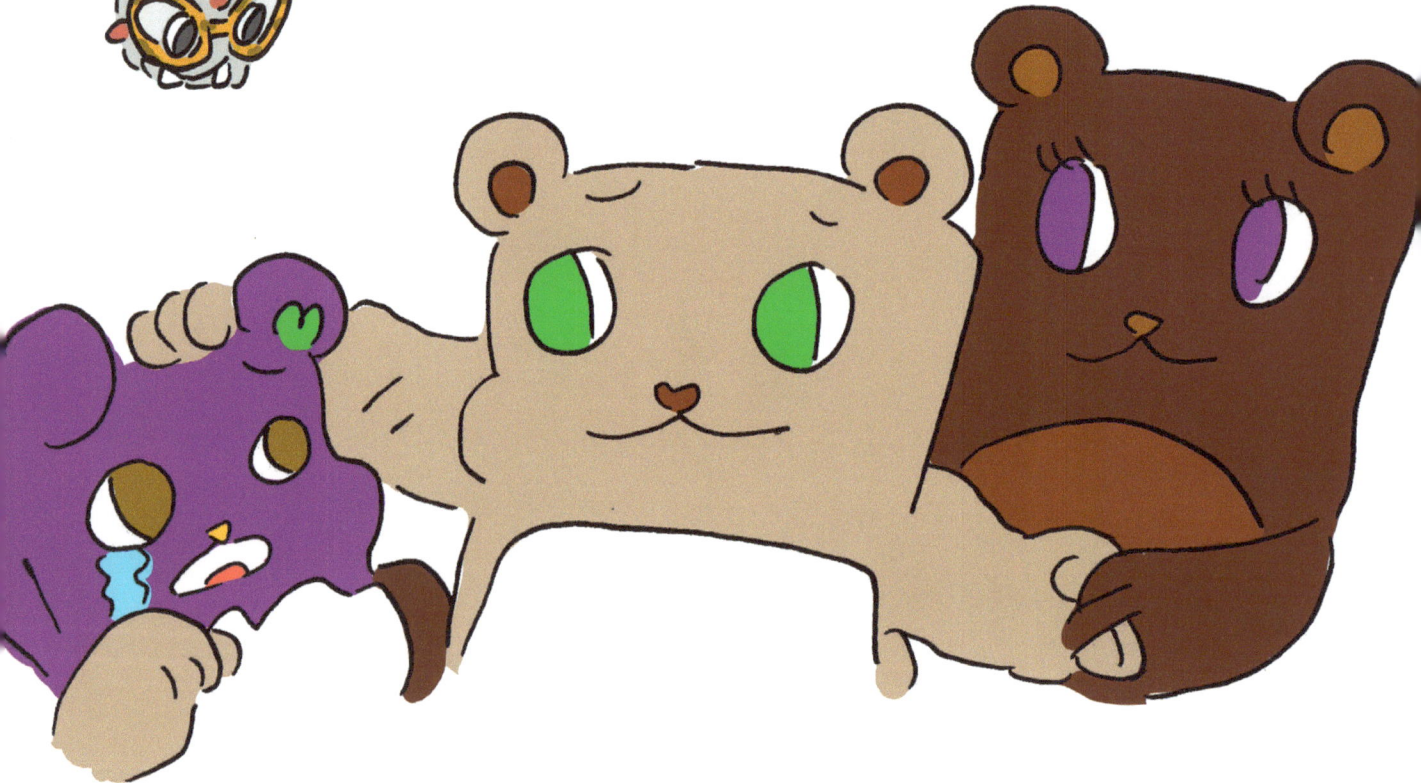

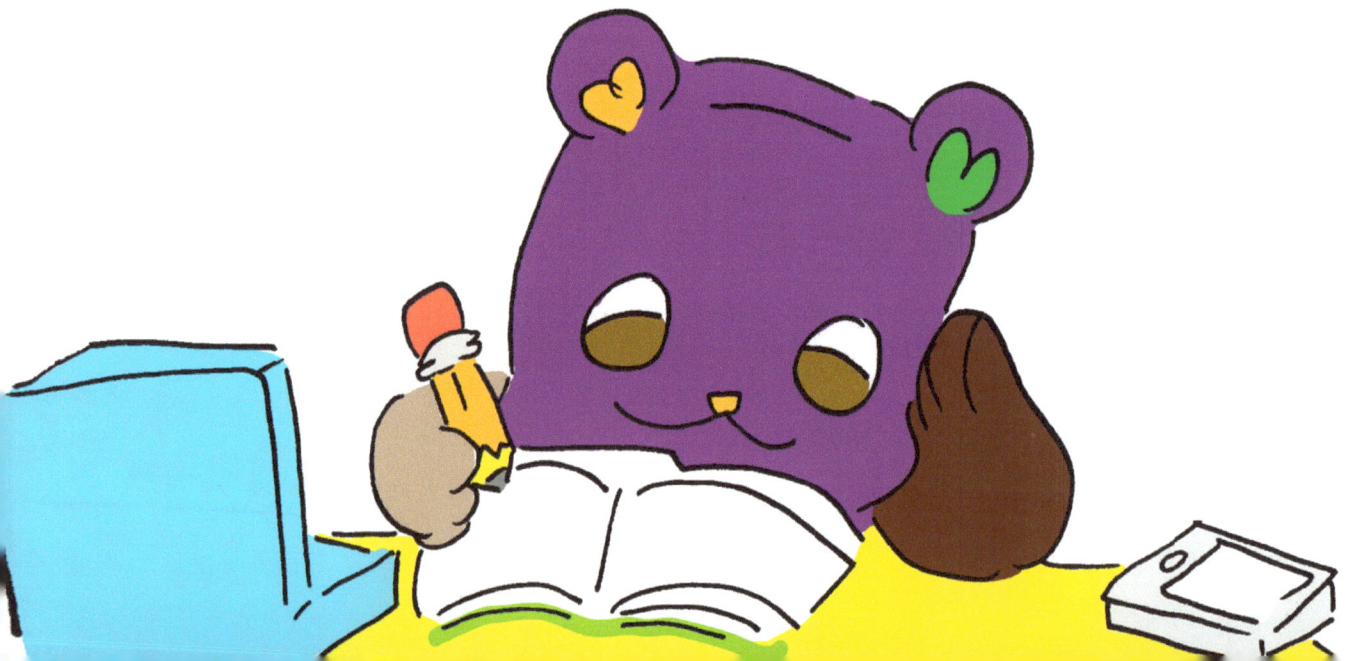

"For family fun, you can sing, dance, draw, and jump rope."

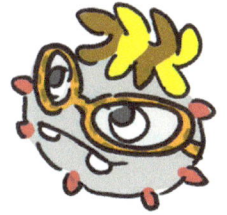

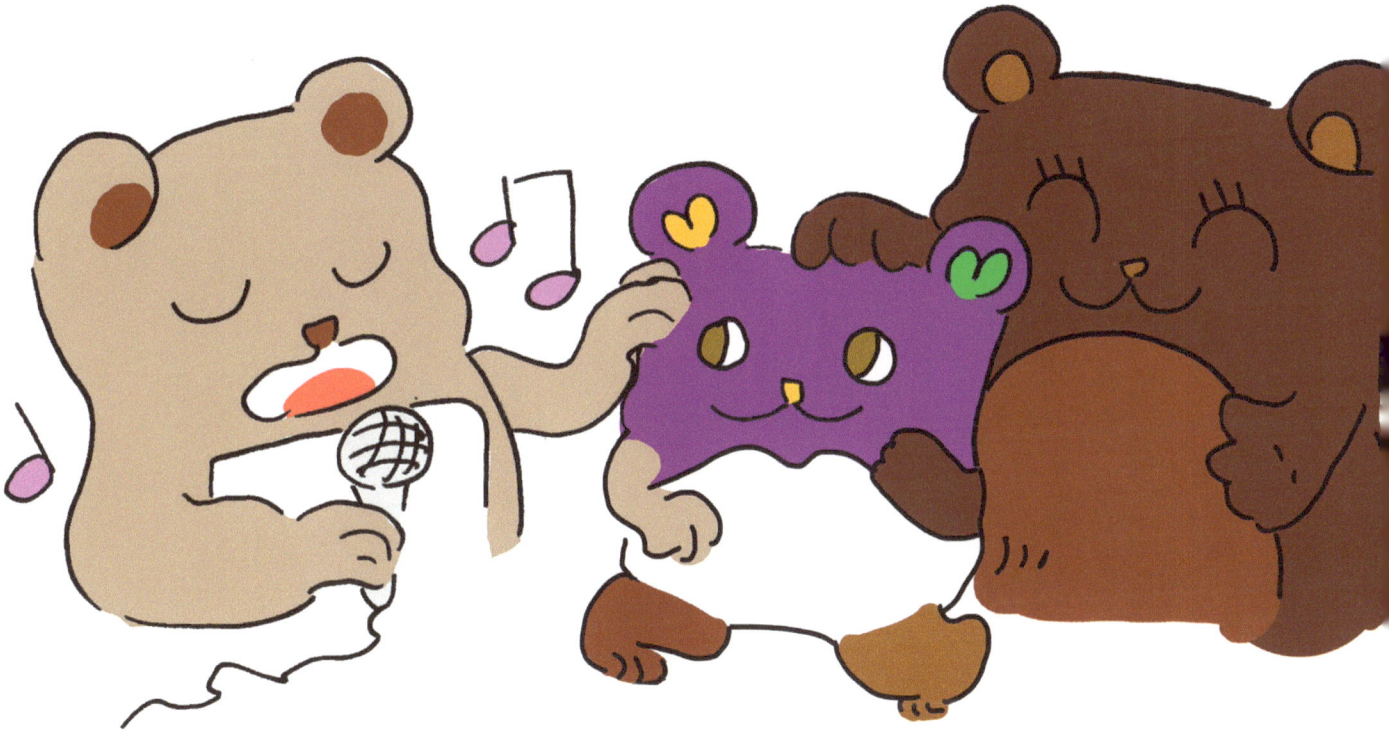

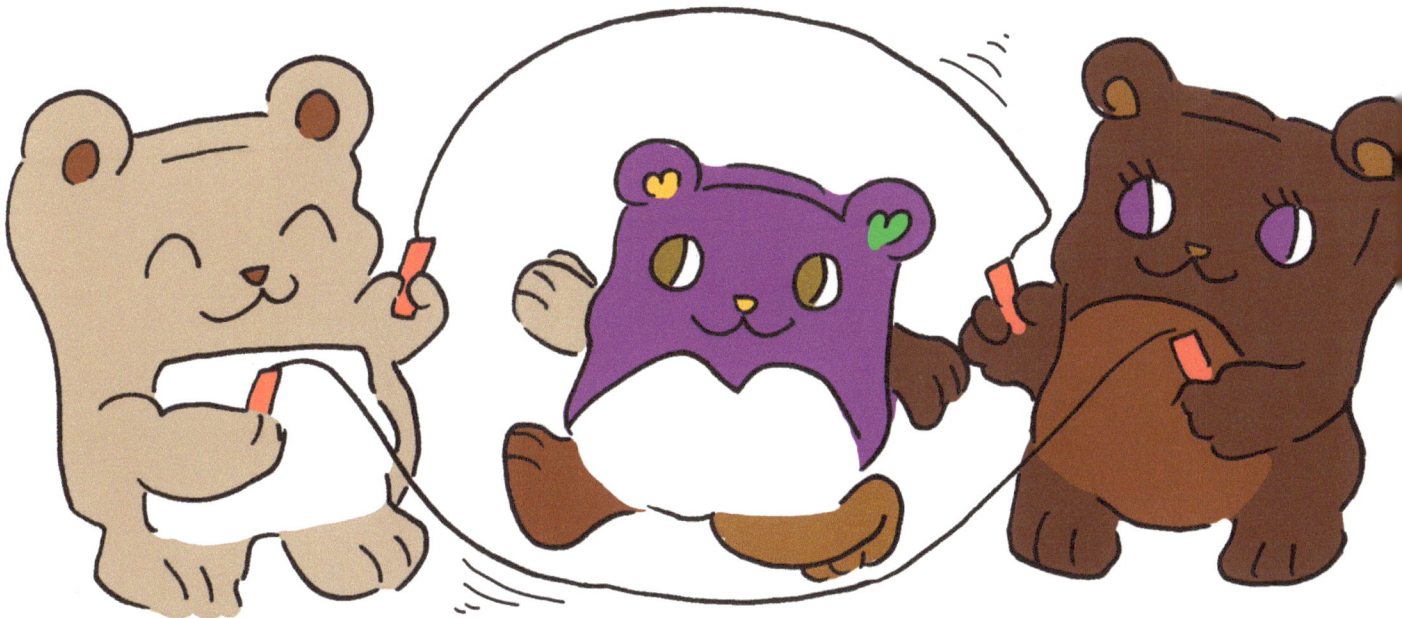

"You can also breathe and stretch with yoga, play board games, and perform magic tricks."

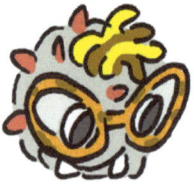

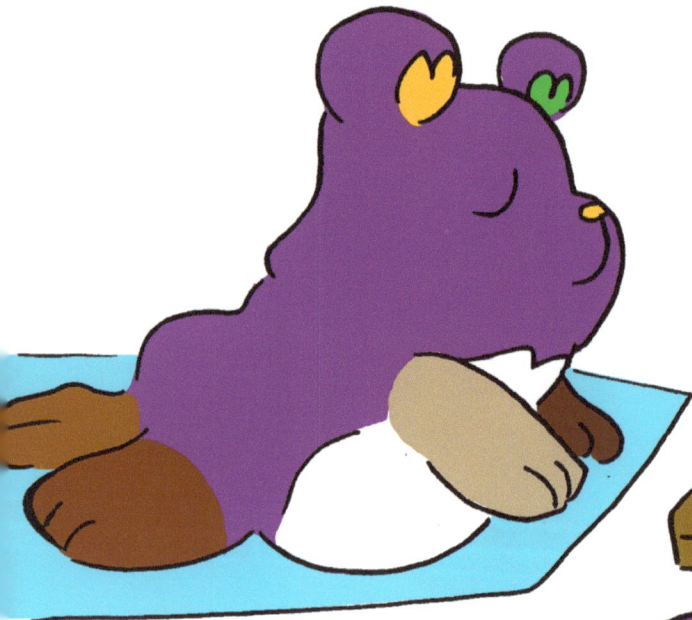

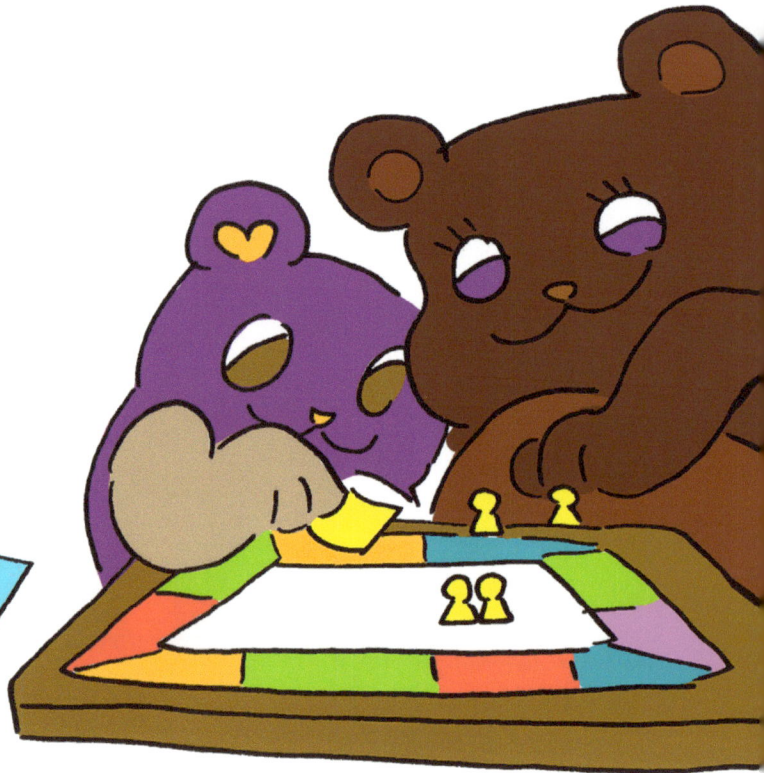

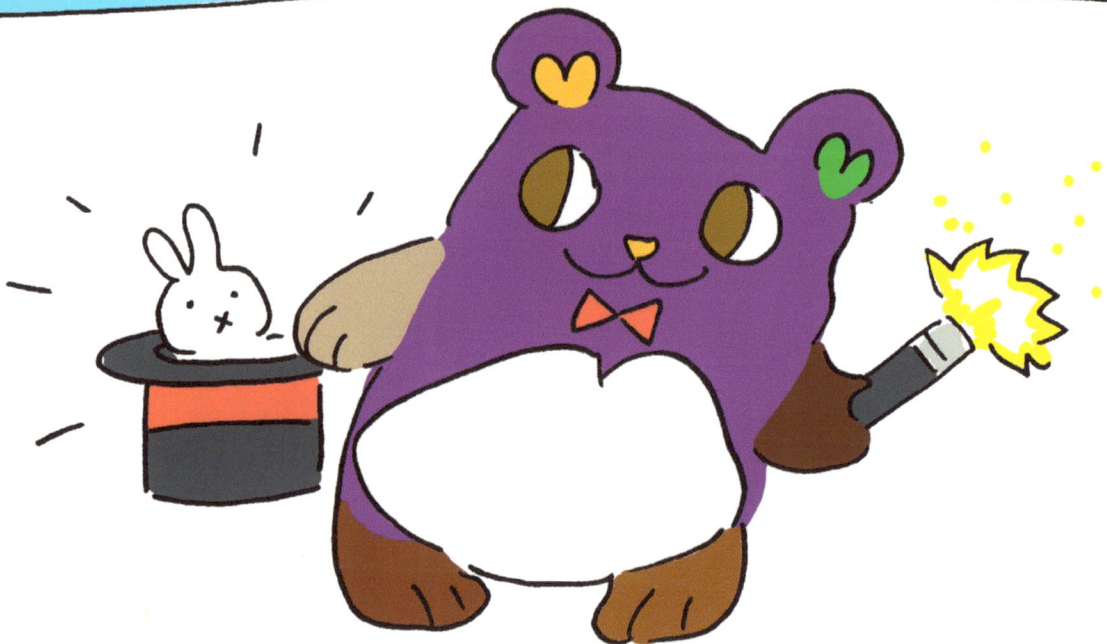

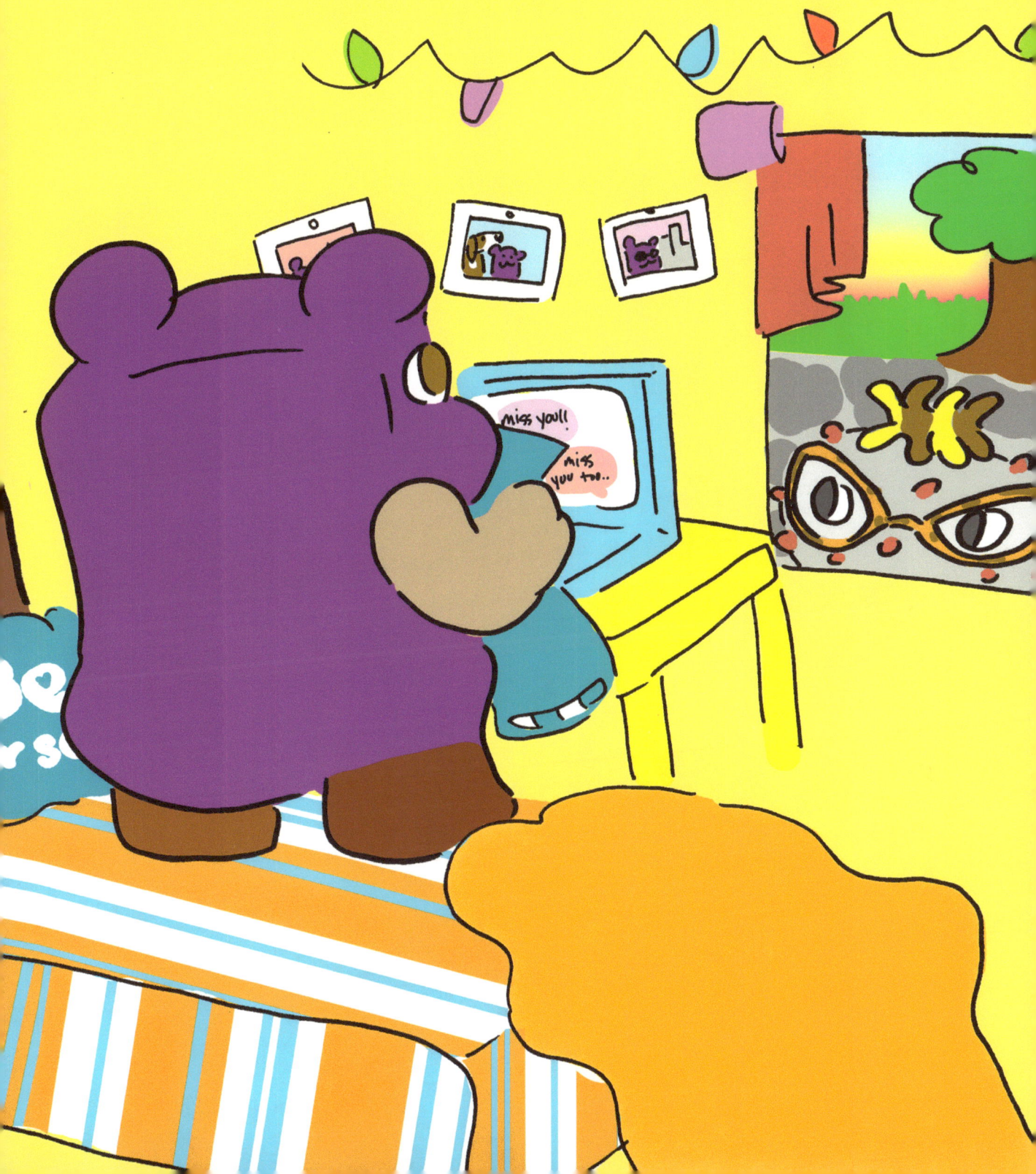

"This sounds so much better than playing with just a stick."

"Yes it does, Tickles! How about this? Remember, you can still call your friends and talk to them too!"

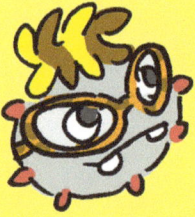

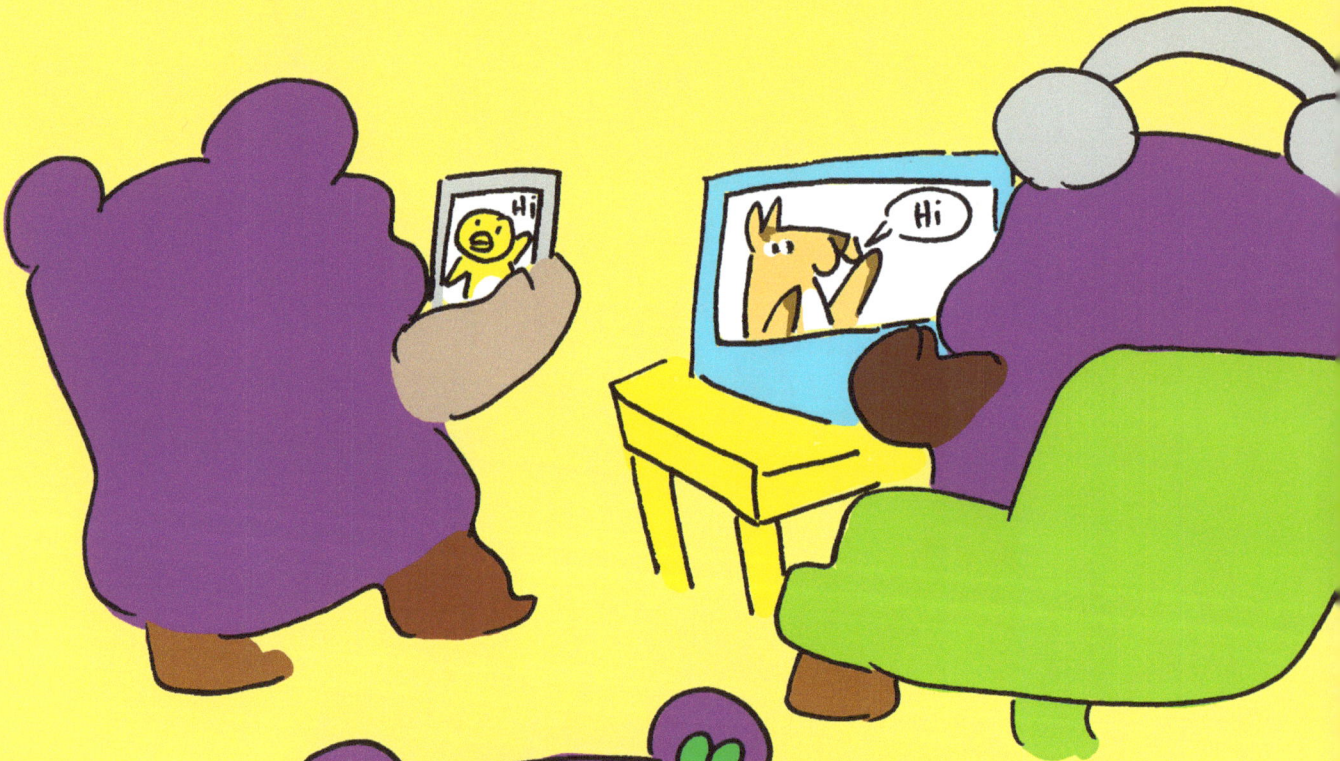

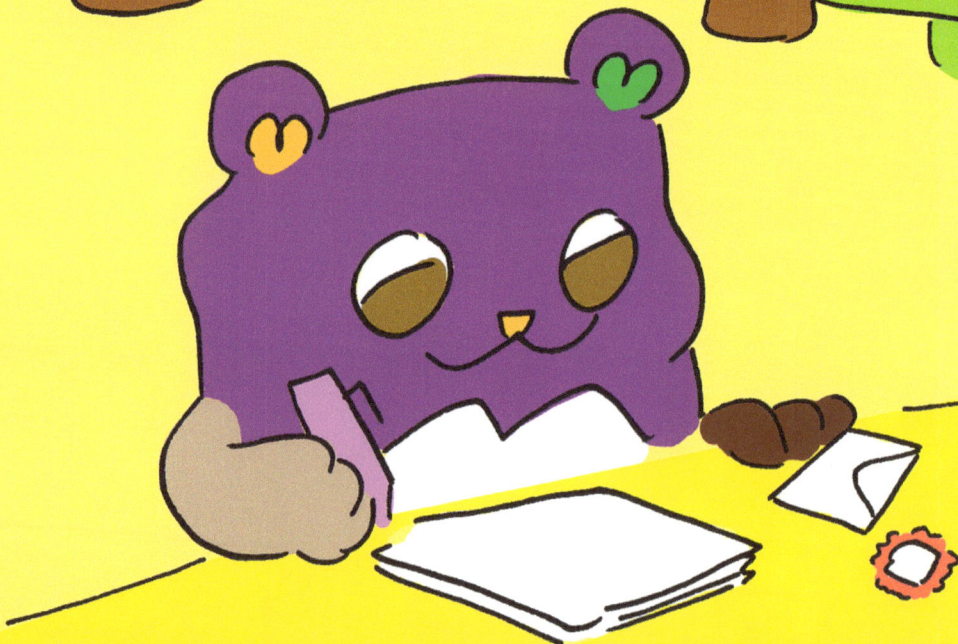

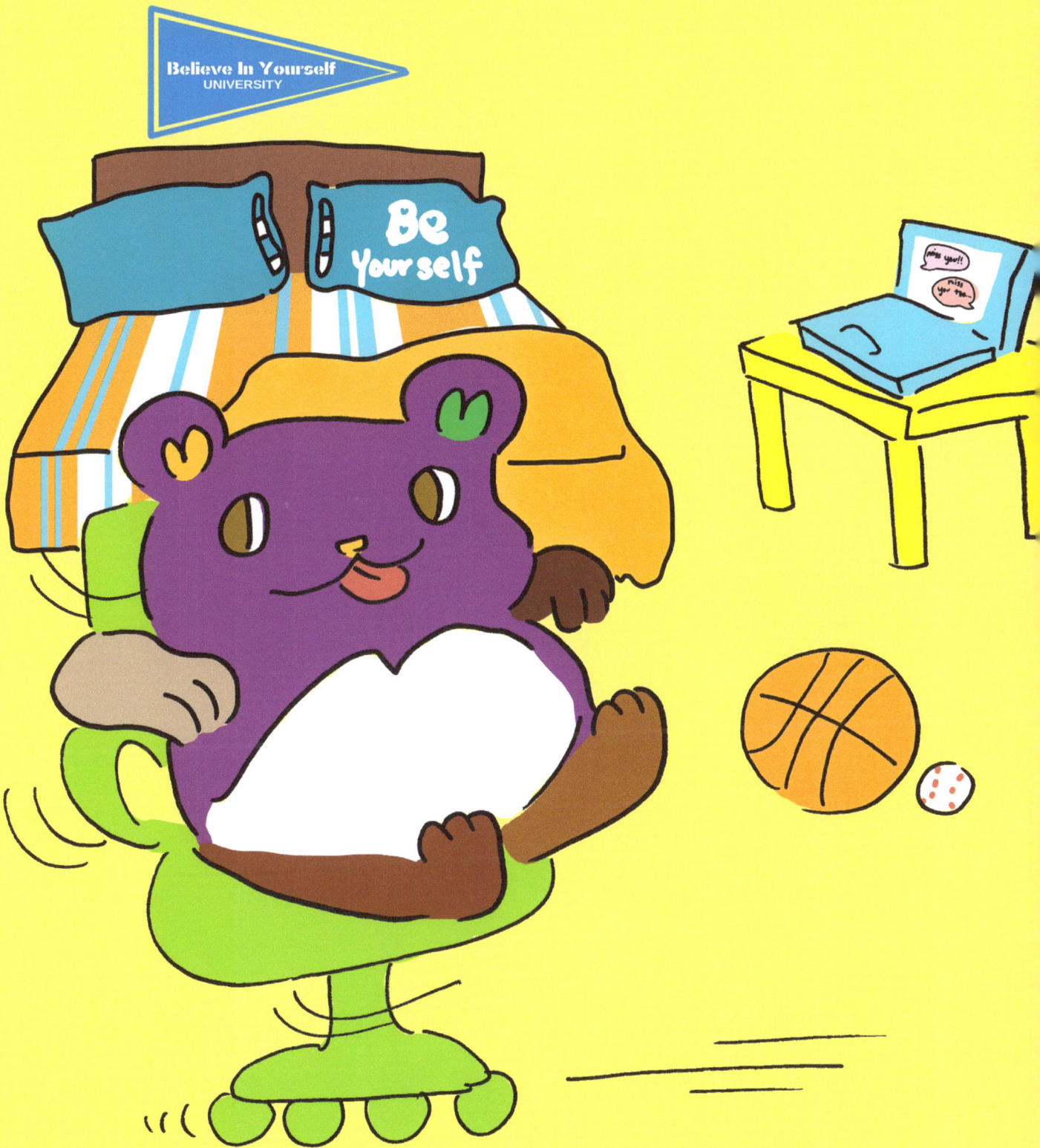

"There are so many entertaining things to do."

"So all of my hopes and dreams won't be ruined either?"

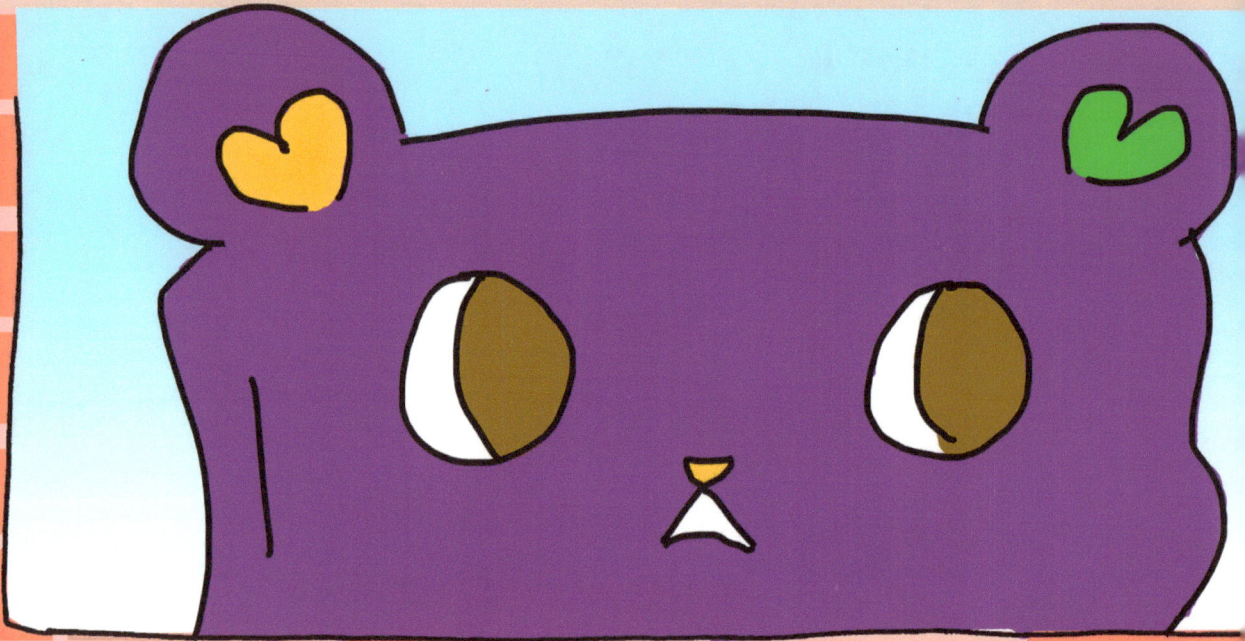

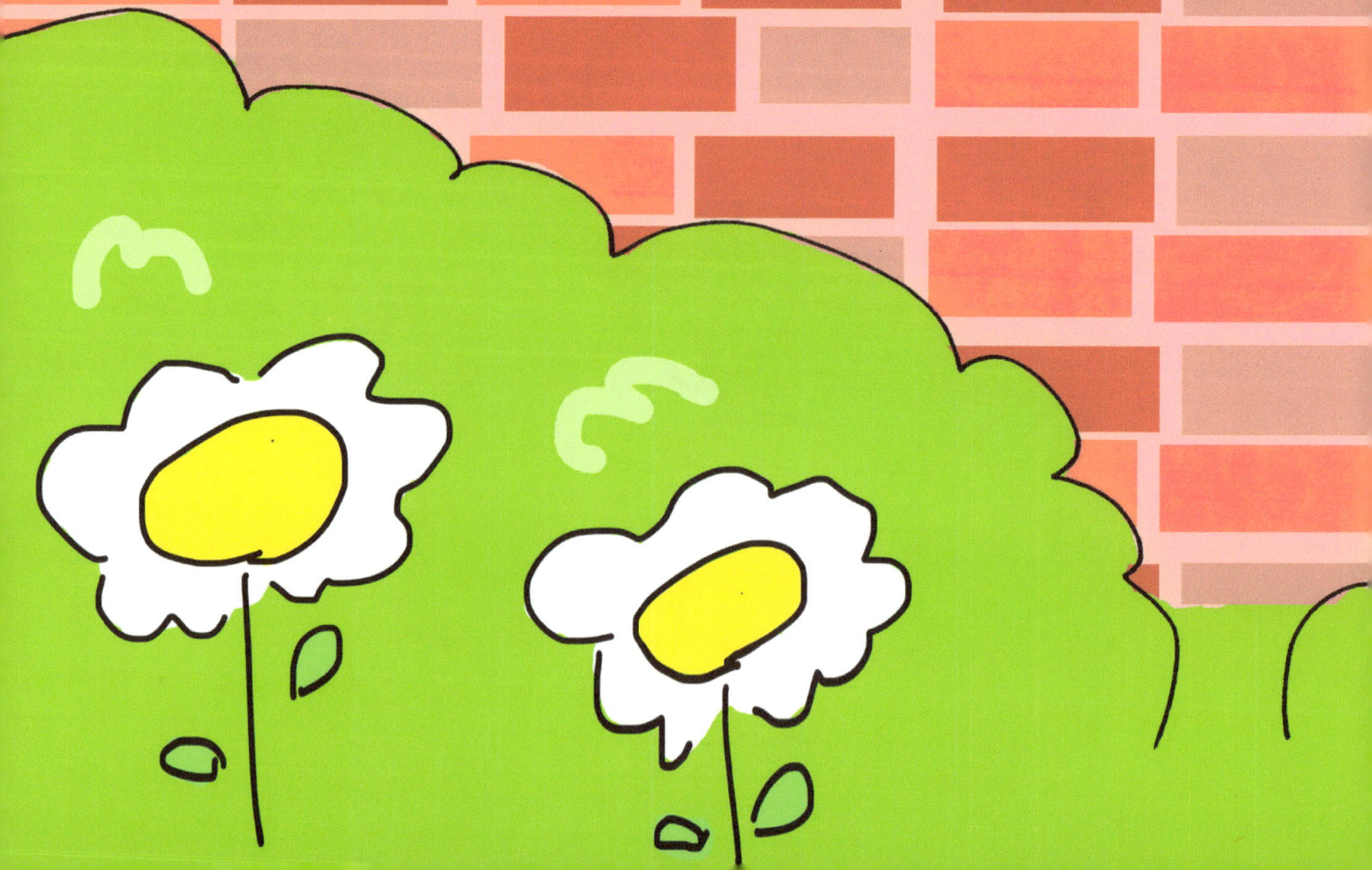

"Oh no, Tickles!"

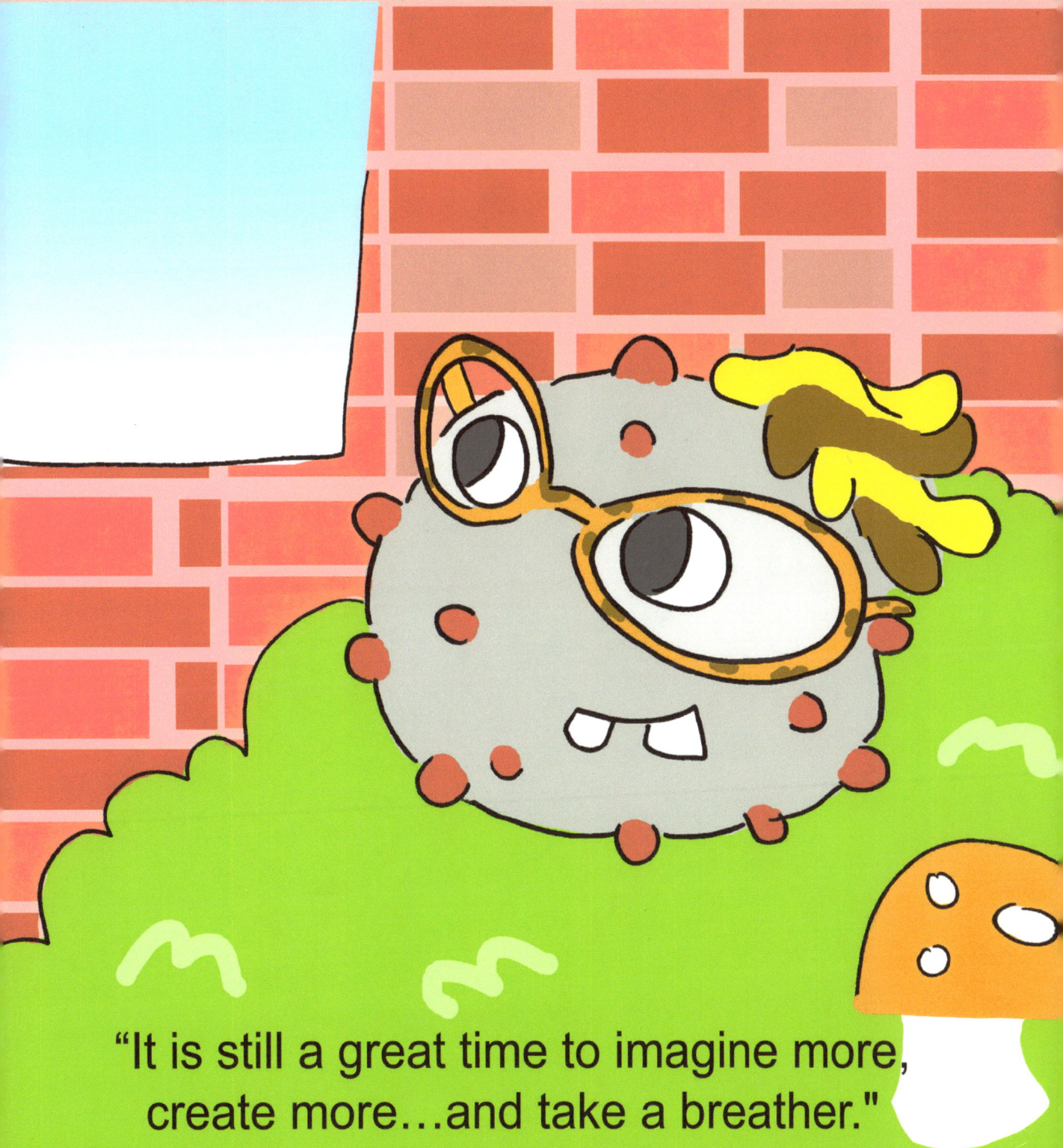

"It is still a great time to imagine more, create more…and take a breather."

"Now do you see why you can't play with me? Your family does not want you to get sick."

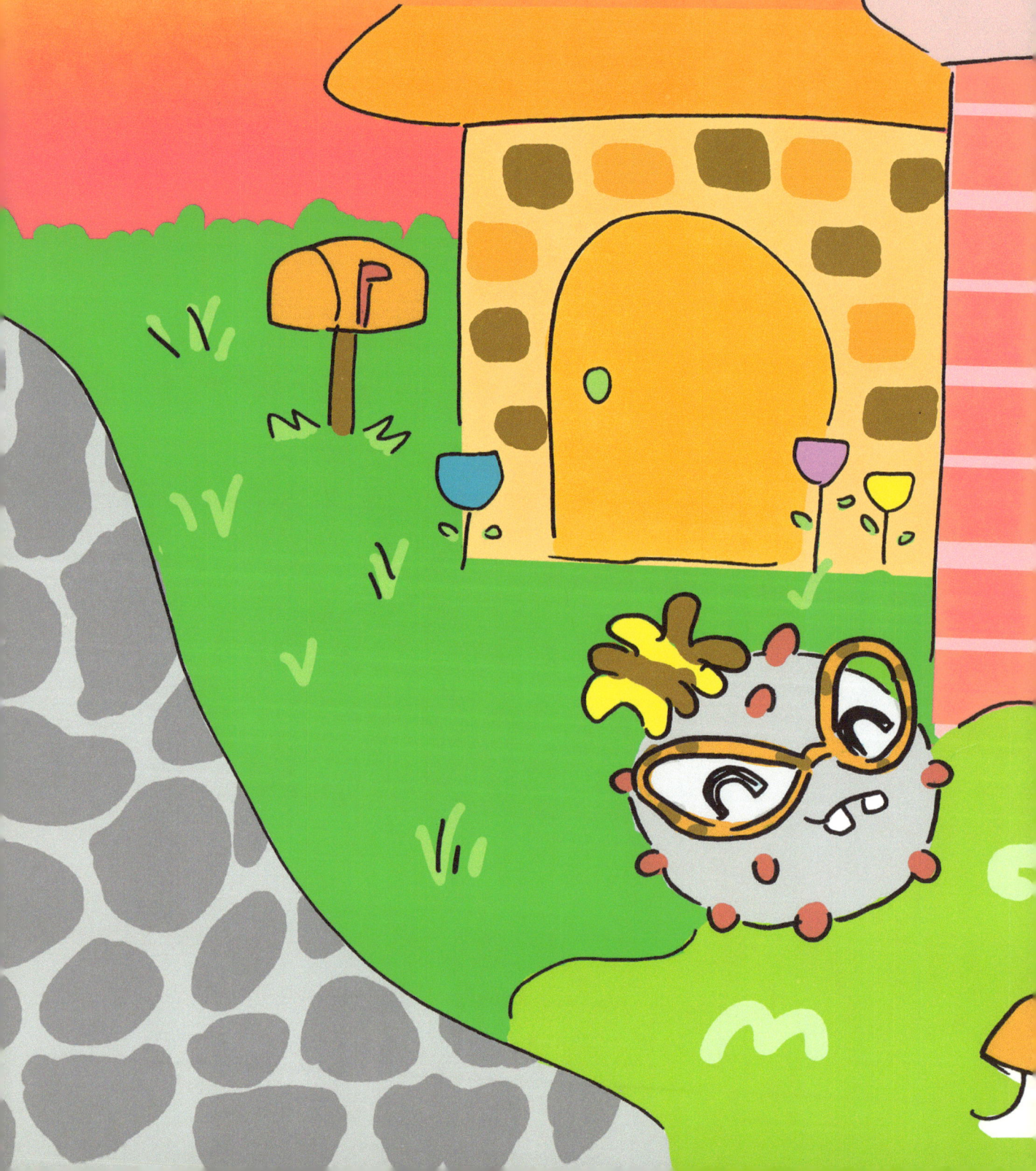

"Yes! And I don't want to feel ick! I understand now what is healthy and safe to do."

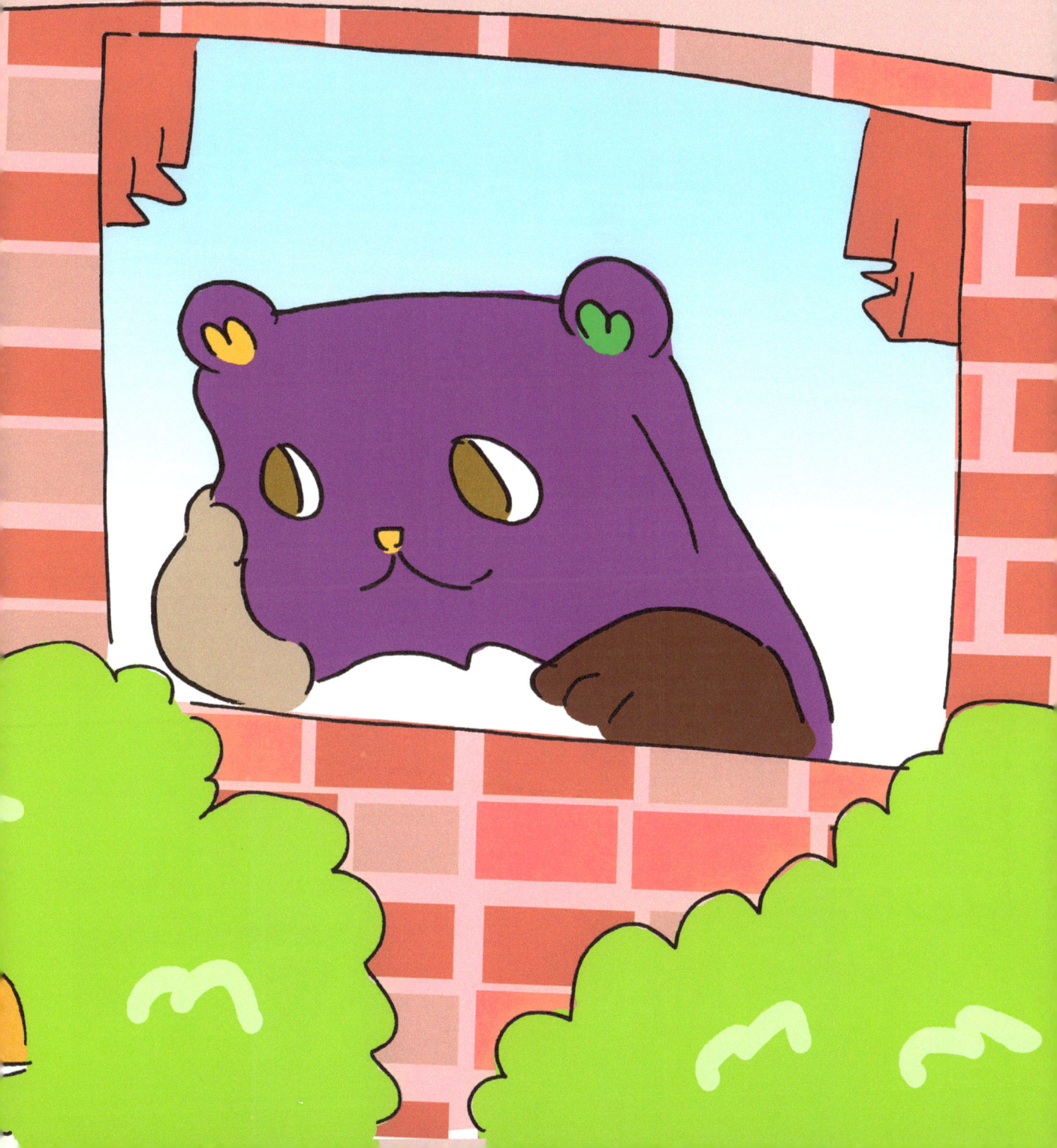

"Good! It won't be much longer before you can play with your friends again, and go back to normal school."

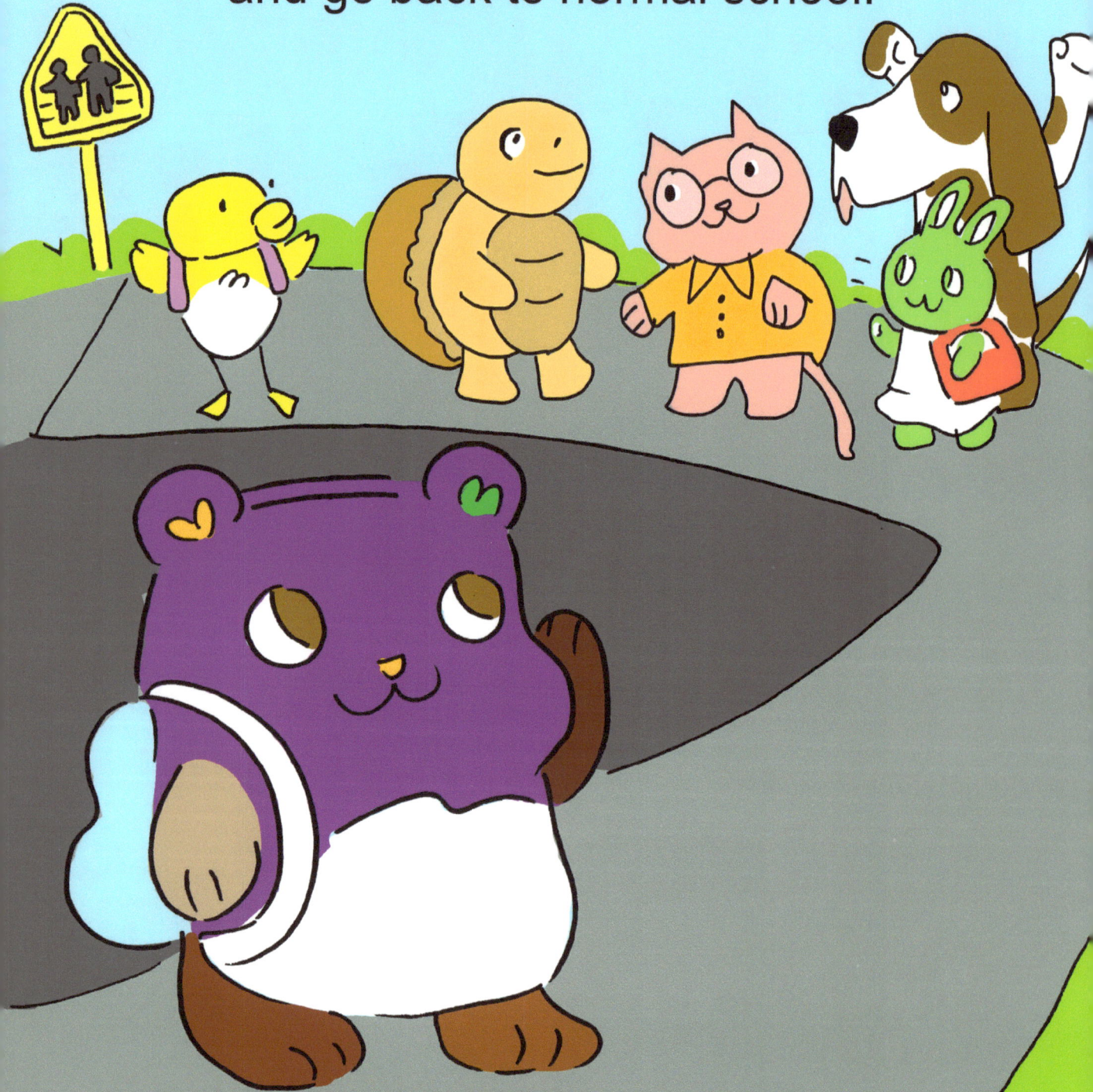

"It's okay to hope for soon."

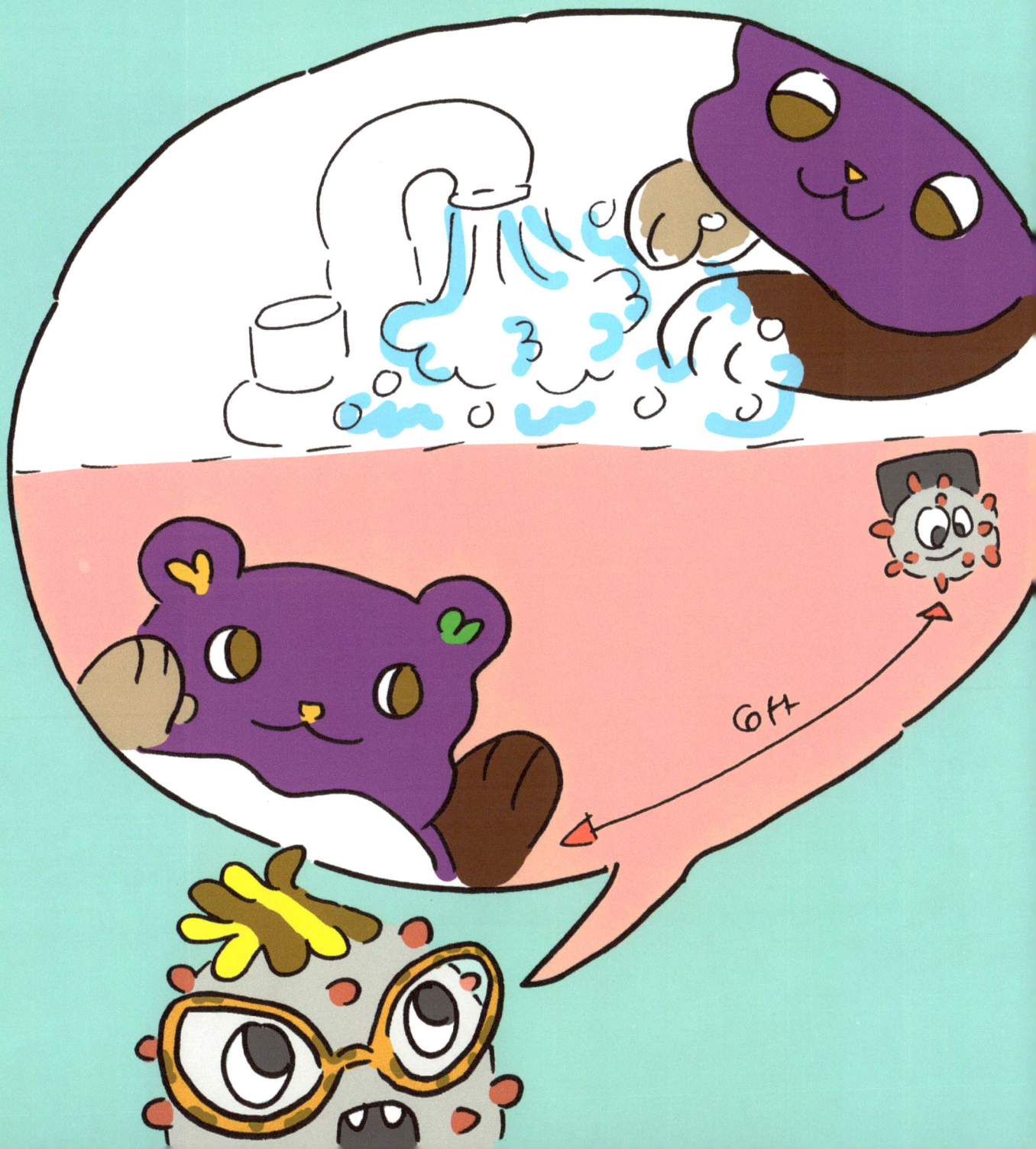

"And don't forget to use your hand washing and social distancing tools."

"I learned so much today,
I'd be happy to use them times two!"

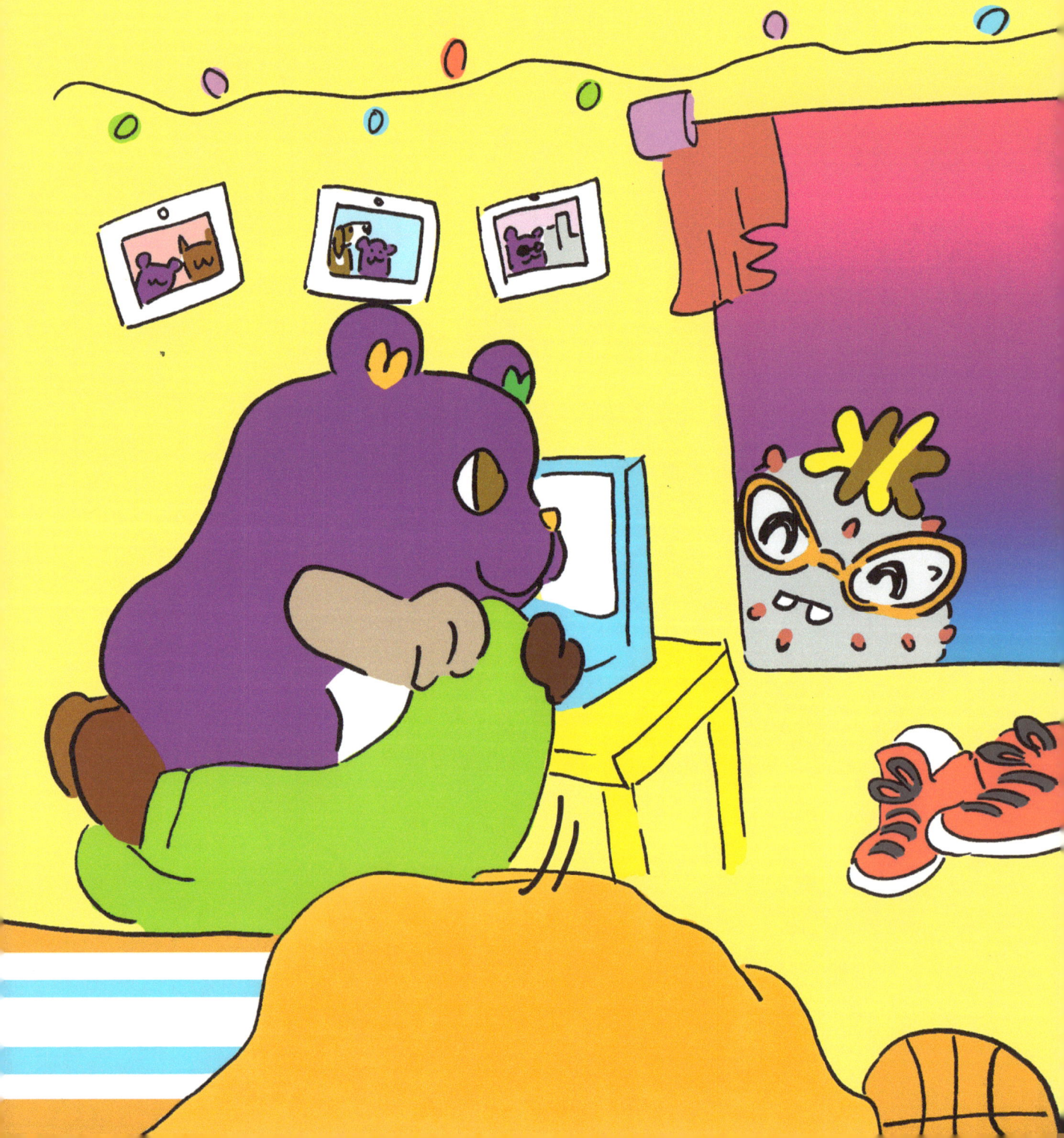

"Thank you for talking with me, Rona.
I have to get ready for bed
before we see the moon."

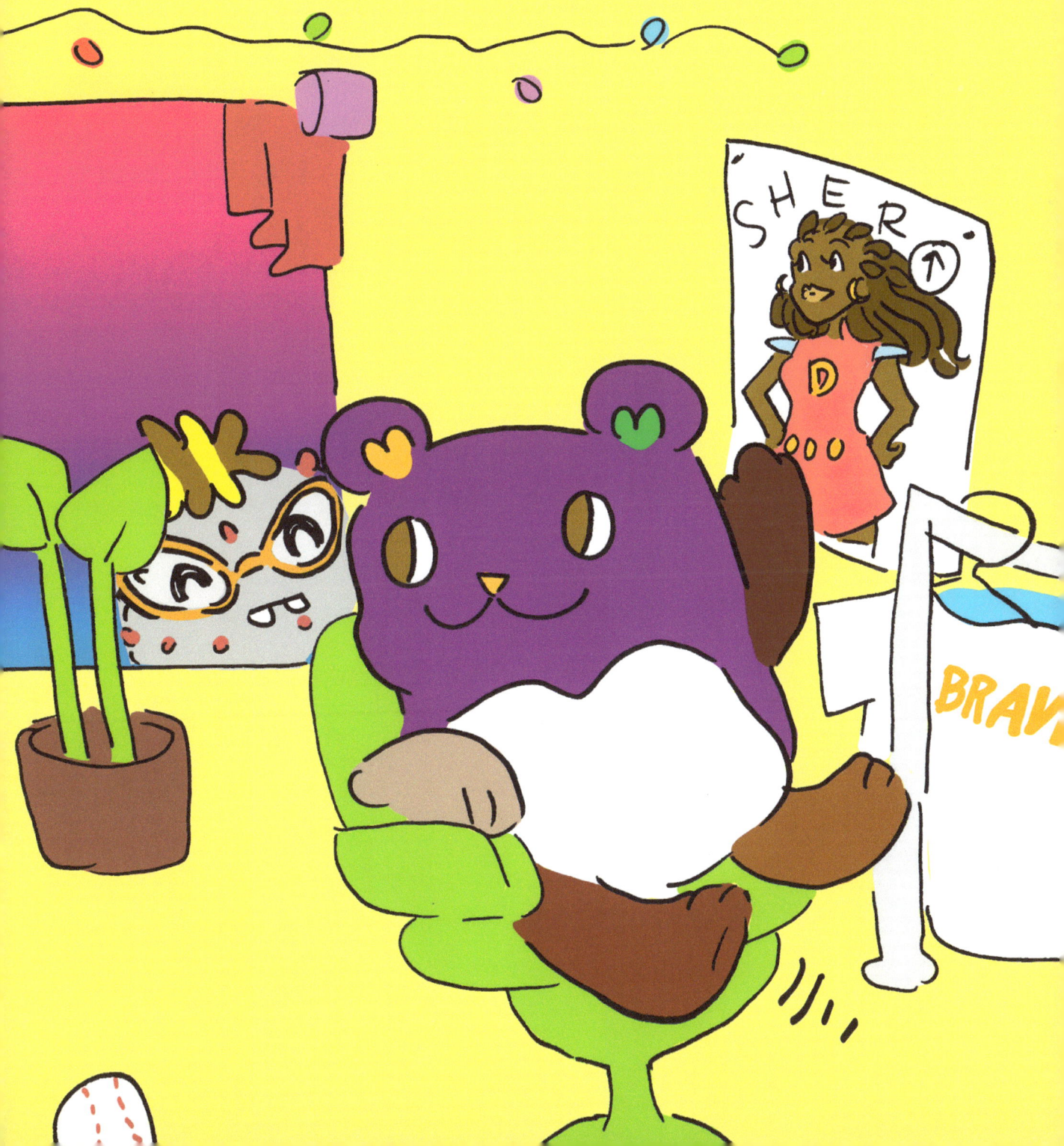

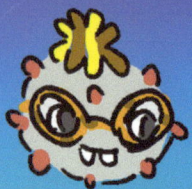

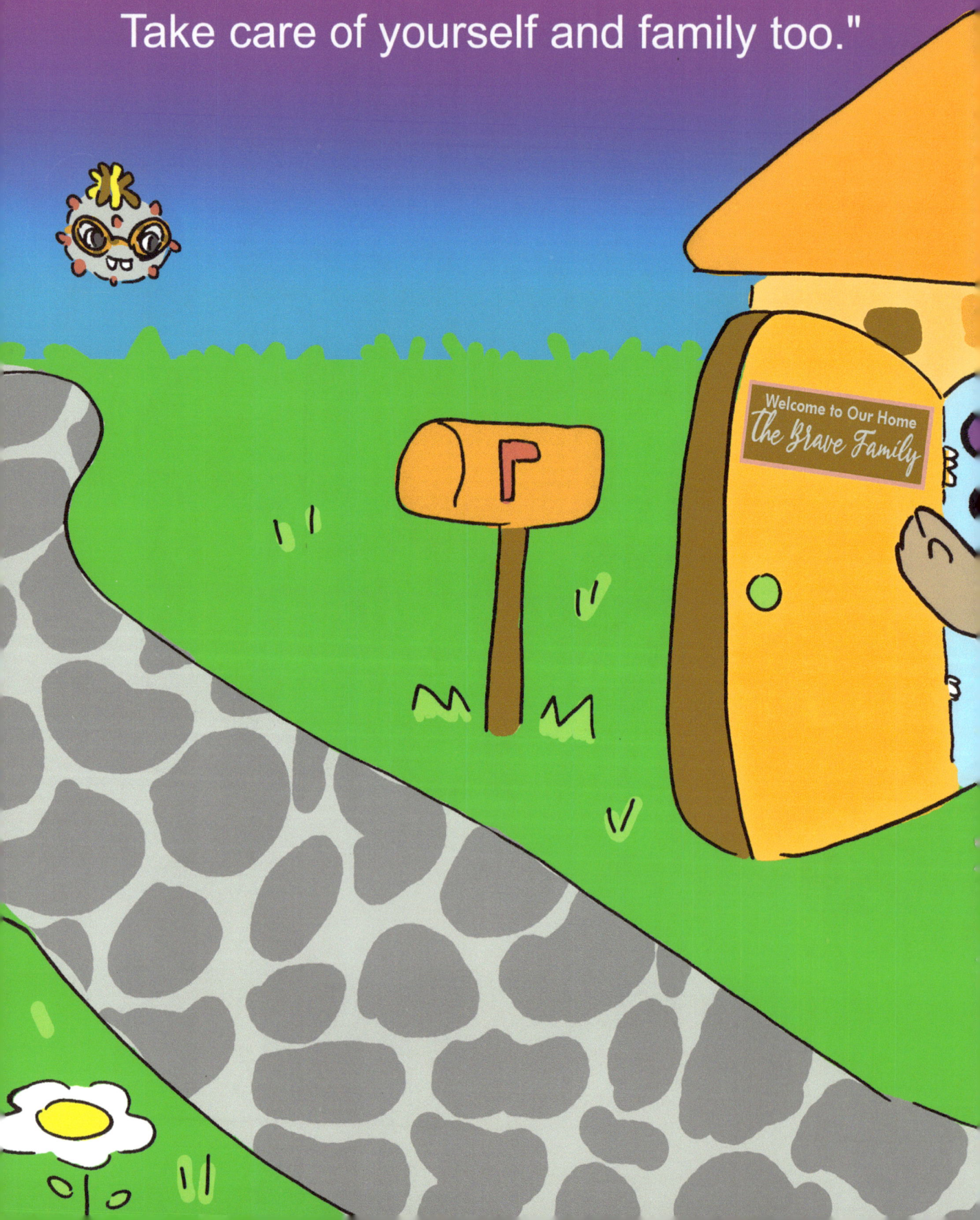

"Goodbye, Rona!
That I will do."

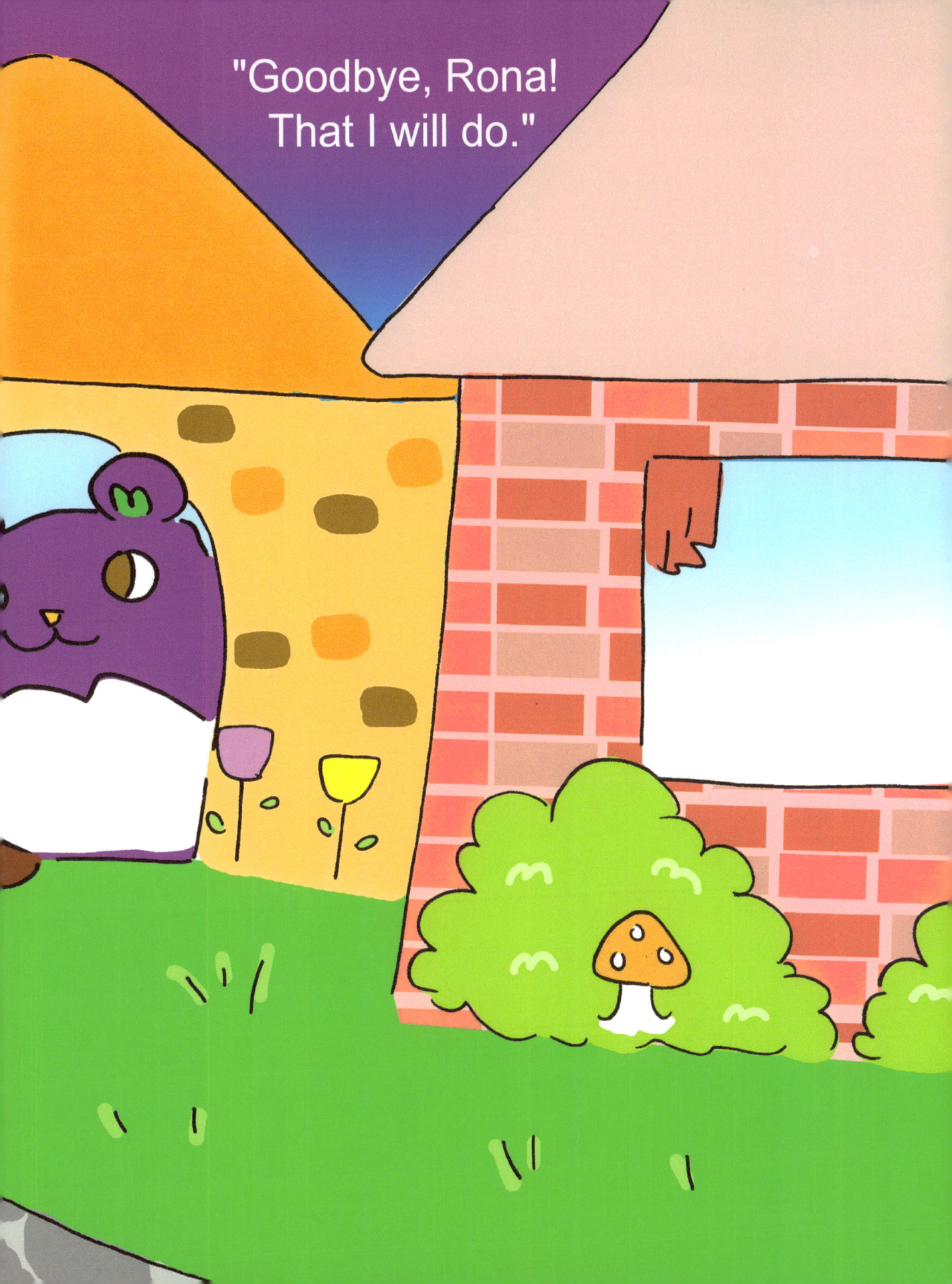

Hey Friends!

To take care of yourself and family too, see the Tickles the Brave Teddy™ "Take Care" Chart on the next pages. Highlighted are ways you and your family may stay safe, healthy, and entertained throughout the pandemic and beyond.

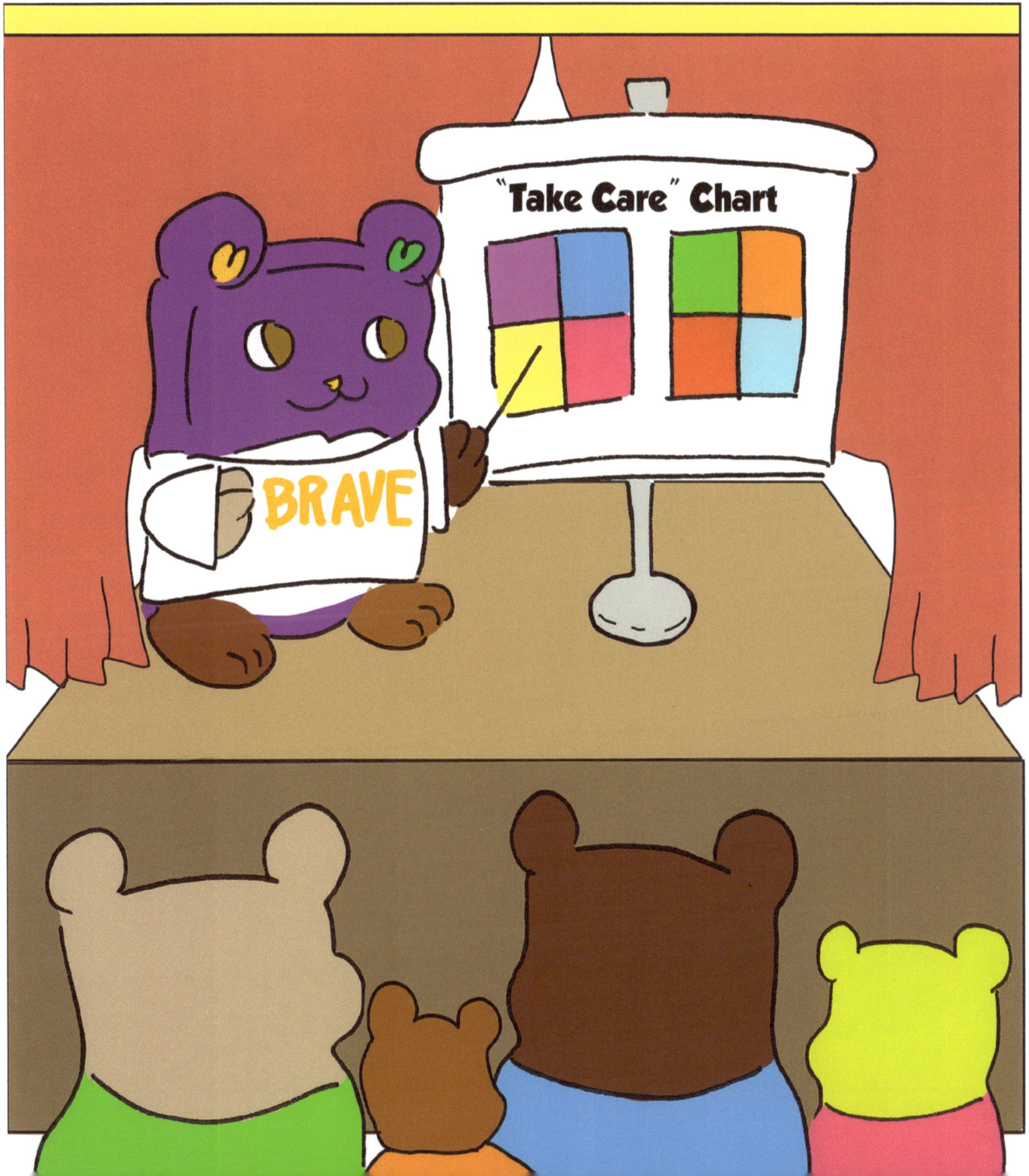

Tickles the Brave Teddy ™

Wash Your Hands

Hand washing with soap and water can help keep our hands clean and reduce spreading germs.

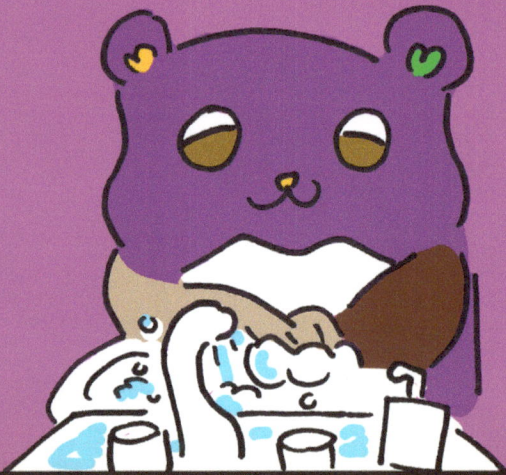

Try New Foods

Adding more fruits and vegetables to our snack and mealtimes can help keep our bodies healthy.

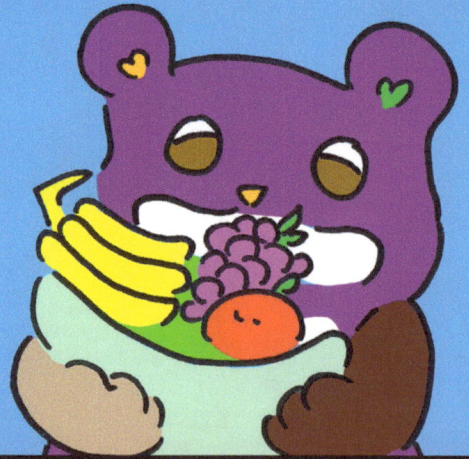

Relax, Get Your Rest

Resting when we need to and getting enough sleep can help keep our minds sharp and ready to learn.

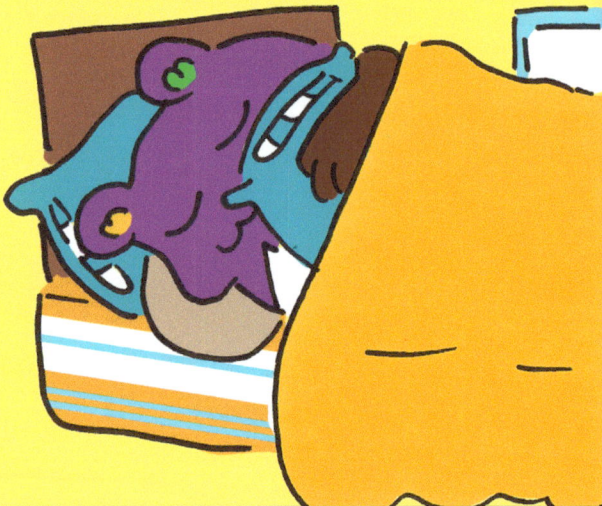

Enjoy Fun Activities

Participating in fun activities we love, or trying new ones, can help increase our creativity.

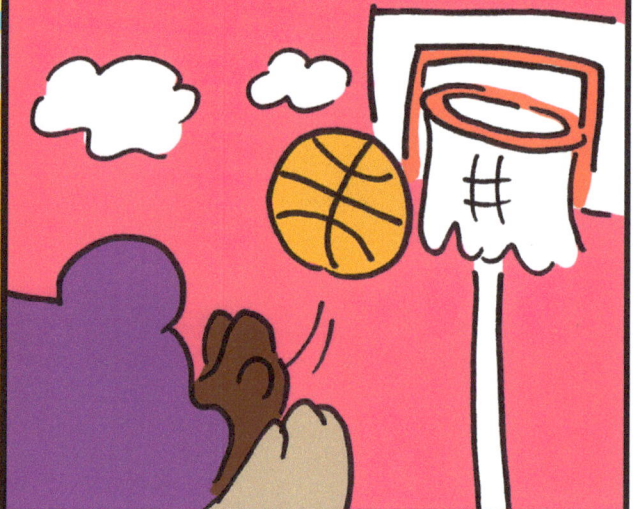

"Take Care" Chart

Move to Music

Engaging in physical activities we love, or trying new ones, can help increase our energy.

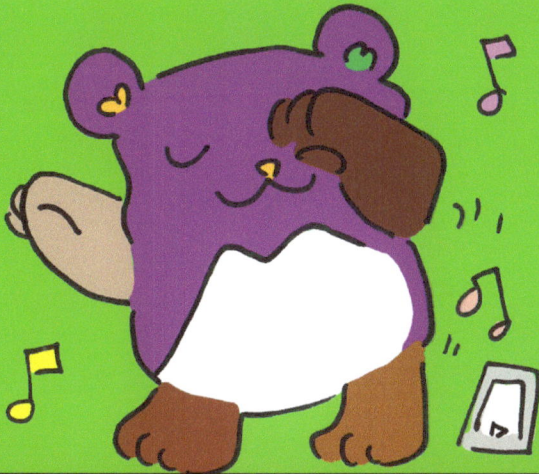

Express Your Feelings

Writing or drawing in a journal can help us express all of our feelings.

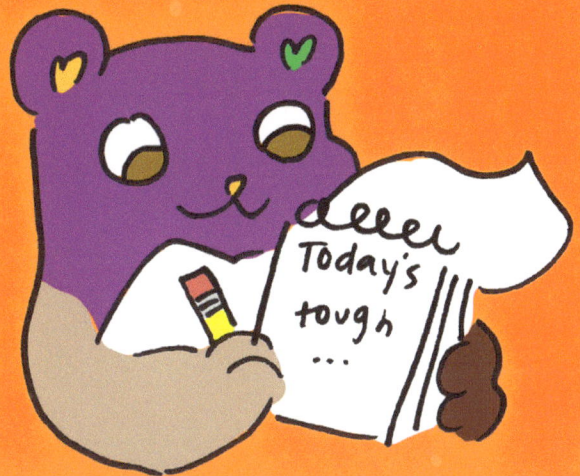

Connect With Family

Spending time with our families can help us connect and become closer.

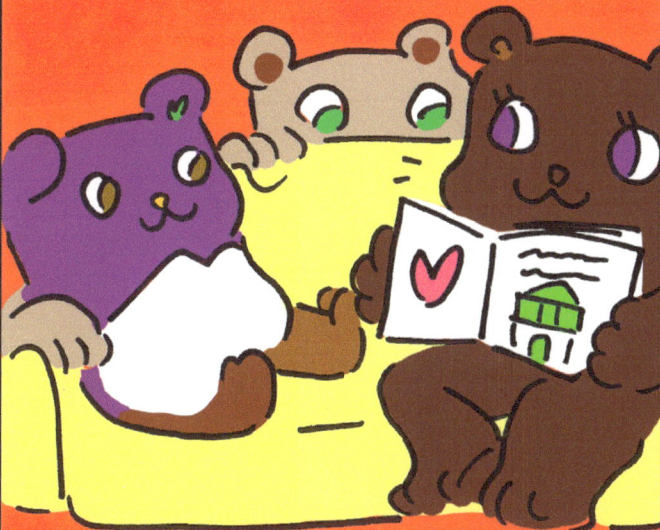

Celebrate With Friends

Talking to our friends can help us get through the times we miss them most.

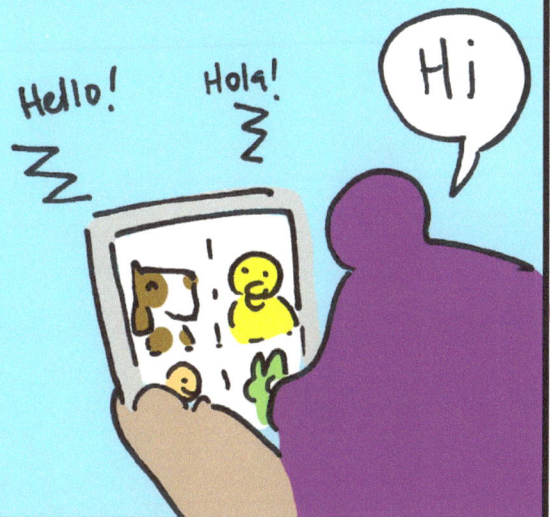

About the Author

Award-winning strategist, speaker and servant leader, Donica' (pronounced: d AA n-ick- uh) is a purpose-driven community investor, and the founder of Complete Package Publishing and Communications, LLC as well as DonicaBEmpowered Global. DonicaBEmpowered Global is a multidimensional personal wellness-empowerment brand, which acts as a "tree of life" for various branch initiatives to reach young professionals, women, and their families. As a seasoned public health professional, she is a researcher, epidemiologist, and educator of all ages, who is passionate about building healthier, wealthier legacies through wellness, empowerment, and philanthropy, globally. Her golden heart for global impact is rooted in the Pear Orchard neighborhood of her hometown, Beaumont, Texas.

Growing up, Donica' collected a variety of stuffed animals. She received her very first teddy bear as a newborn. It was the comfort and joy these brought her, which inspired the book character, Tickles the Brave Teddy™. As a child, she pretended to be a teacher, and shared many lessons with her stuffed animal "students". Her collection grew to include approximately 200 stuffed animals, overtime. They have since been donated for other children to love and enjoy.

Brave Like Me! Courageous Lessons About the COVID-19 Coronavirus and Healthy Coping for Children and Families Anytime is her debut picture book.

About the Illustrator

Jean Marie Munson has been drawing since she was a kid, and is happy she is an adult drawing illustrations for all ages! She's a podcaster, teacher, and dog mom rolled into one. Comics are her first love and then her husband, but they are totally interchangeable day-to-day. She hopes that kids keep drawing and adults return to being kids at heart.

About the Publisher

Complete Package Publishing and Communications, LLC (CPPC) is a community-driven, publishing and communications firm. Operating using a social justice lens, we aim to increase access to family health literature, narrow gaps in health communication and literacy, and promote diversity and inclusion in media and beyond. We believe that "no society is complete without a collective voice, which oppresses none™"—hence the company name. We empower diverse communities to collectively cultivate healthier and more equitable legacies for all families. We envision a nation and world where health equity is achieved through innovative and inclusive partnerships, literary works and communication strategy.

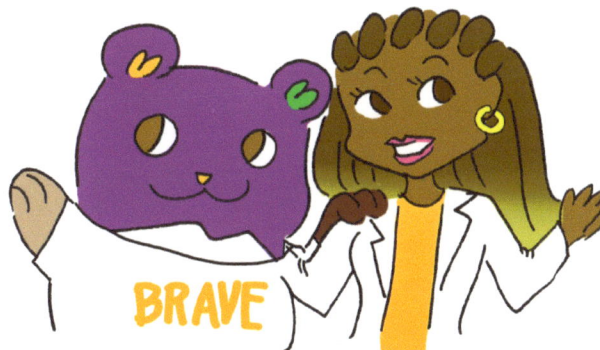

Thanks for reading.
Take care.
Family health is LIT !

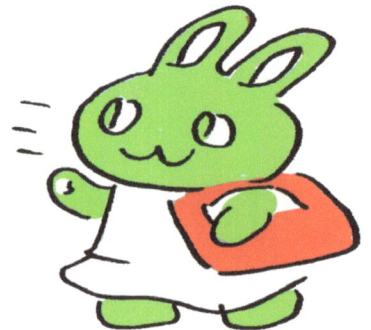

www.ingramcontent.com/pod-product-compliance
Lightning Source LLC
Chambersburg PA
CBHW041542260326
41914CB00015B/1520